WHAT TO EAT NOW

The Cancer Lifeline Cookbook

*and easy-to-use nutrition guide to delicious
and healthy eating for cancer patients,
survivors, and caregivers*

by Rachel Keim with Ginny Smith

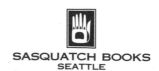

SASQUATCH BOOKS
SEATTLE

Printed in the United States of America.
Published by Sasquatch Books
Distributed in Canada by Raincoast Books Ltd.

Cover and interior illustrations by Susan Olivier-Hirasawa
Design and typesetting by Susan Olivier-Hirasawa

Library of Congress Cataloging in Publication Data
Keim, Rachel
    What to Eat Now: the Cancer Lifeline cookbook and easy-to-use nutririon guide to
delicious and healthy eating for cancer patients, survivors, and caregivers / by Rachel
Kiem with Ginny Smith.
      p.   cm.
    Includes index.
    ISBN 1-57061-073-8
    1. Cancer—Nutritional aspects. 2. Cancer—Diet therapy.
I. Smith, Ginny. II. Title.
RC268.45.K45   1996
616.99'40654—cd20   96-3934

Sasquatch Books
1008 Western Avenue
Seattle, Washington 98104
(206) 467-4300

Dedication

Cancer Lifeline's *What to Eat Now* is dedicated to Dorothy S. O'Brien, a cancer survivor who created her own informal, mini Cancer Lifeline before she even knew that Cancer Lifeline existed.

Dorothy and her husband, Bob—her Caregiver Extraordinaire during her illness—firmly believe that good nutrition played a significant role in Dorothy's complete recovery, and they have generously provided the financial support needed to publish this book.

Thank you, Dorothy and Bob!

Acknowledgments

Cancer Lifeline owes a large debt of gratitude to the numerous individuals whose personal and professional expertise and insights, long hours of effort, and boundless enthusiasm have helped us take a great idea and make it a reality.

At the top of our list are Rachel Keim and Ginny Smith—who devoted month after month to planning, researching, writing and rewriting the manuscript—and their families, friends, and co-workers who were patient and supportive during those sometimes trying times.

We would also like to extend special thanks to Susan Olivier-Hirasawa, designer of the book; Jennifer McCord, publishing consultant; Lindsey McDonald, marketing consultant; Frances Albrecht, MS, CN, nutrition consultant; Suzzanne Myer, MS, RD, Assistant Professor, Bastyr University; Ellen Zahlis, RN, MN; Marianne Sterling, RN; Barney McCallum; Marilyn Clement; and Marnie Keough. Their professional expertise, talent, enthusiasm, and dedication have played a major role in bringing this book to fruition.

Chefs and restaurants who have contributed recipes to our book include Kerry Sear, executive chef, Four Seasons Hotel; Ludger Szmania, chef, Szmania; Jim Watkins, chef, Plenty Café and Fine Foods; Alvin Binyua, chef, Ponti Seafood Grill; Jacques Boiroux, chef, formerly co-owner of Le Tastevin and now food consultant to Queen Anne Thriftway and KIRO TV; Todo Loco; Fresh Ideas; and Pasta and Company—all of Seattle, Washington.

In addition, we are grateful to all the individuals who reviewed *What to Eat Now* for us and offered suggestions. Health care professionals include Rick Clarfeld, MD, breast surgeon; Jay Klarnet, MD, oncologist; Jack Leversee, MD, family practitioner; Dan Labriola, ND; Mary Ellen Shands, RN, MN; Ann Fote, RN; Lynn Behar, MSW, patient oncology; Sandra Johnson, MSW, supervisor, cancer support services; Judith Jones, BS, cancer education specialist; Marilyn Ward, RD; Shirley Stensland, RD, MS, nutrition consultant; and Susan Goedde, MSW, patient oncology.

Cancer Lifeline board members, Friends of Cancer Lifeline members, and volunteers who reviewed the book include: Carol Jean Berg, Shirley Brandenburg, Dodie Capeloto, Mary Clarfeld, Pat Clemence, Nancy B. Evans, Janet Hahn, RN, Catherine Hennum, Pam Hill, Donna Neve, Dorothy O'Brien, Connie Pious, and Marianne Sterling, RN.

Recipes were tried by survivors and their family members, Cancer Lifeline board members, Friends of Cancer Lifeline members, and Cancer Lifeline staff members. Staff members, of course, have played a major role in the development of *What to Eat Now,* and we extend special thanks to each of them. We would like to thank Gary Luke, Joan Gregory, and all the people at Sasquatch Books for their cooperation and support.

And finally, we would like to thank all the cancer survivors—as well as their caregivers, family members, and friends—whose desire to make healthy nutritional choices, improve their sense of well-being, and take more control over their lives provided the inspiration for this book in the first place.

DISCLAIMER

Cancer Lifeline makes no warranty of any nature, express or implied, concerning the effectiveness of the recipes or diet suggestions included in this publication as a means to prevent or cure any form of cancer.

CONTENTS

INTRODUCTION

It is generally accepted that 30 percent of all cancers are linked to diet. What's more, what we eat may have a significant impact on our ability to fight cancer once it has developed. The connection between diet and cancer has been formally recognized by both the Surgeon General of the United States and the National Academy of Sciences. The National Cancer Institute has formed a division specifically designed to study the various known anticancer substances in food. The American Dietetic Association supports the use of nutrients to help prevent cancer. In 1980 the National Cancer Institute commissioned a comprehensive study of scientific information on the relation between diet, nutrition, and cancer. Evidence emerged suggesting that dietary patterns influence cancers of most major sites and that proper diet eventually could reduce the incidence of cancer by approximately one-third.

Because good nutrition is so important before, during, and after treatment, *What to Eat Now* is primarily for people living with cancer. However, this book is also intended for anyone interested in a health-conscious diet. It sets the stage for a healthier lifestyle from which we all can benefit.

We at Cancer Lifeline decided to create *What to Eat Now* for a number of reasons. As you have already read, accumulating data supports the link between diet and cancer. Yet, cancer survivors have been encouraged to maintain their weight at all costs—even if that means eating a high-fat, high-sugar, low-fiber, low-nutrient diet. While this may be necessary in some cases, current thinking tells us that it's often possible to maintain weight on a low-fat, high-fiber, nutrient-rich diet that simultaneously boosts the body's ability to fight disease. When, in 1994, Cancer Lifeline couldn't find any books that provided a comprehensive description of how to do that, we decided to create our own.

So *what can you expect from* **What to Eat Now?**

▲ Easy-to-understand descriptions of the key components of good nutrition, including the Top 10 "Super Foods"—which may protect and fight against cancer.

▲ Practical, easy-to-implement suggestions for incorporating healthy eating into your lifestyle.

▲ A variety of recipes for great-tasting, nutritious dishes that are quick and easy to make—even if you're a novice in the kitchen.

▲ A helpful resource for caregivers who are trying *so hard* to make meals that are "right" and healthy for the cancer patient. Many of these caregivers are spouses who have limited cooking experience.

▲ Suggestions for reducing the side effects of cancer treatment.

▲ Help in improving your quality of life and your sense of well-being and control.

It is important to remember that diet alone is not the sole cause of any cancer, nor is a nutritious diet alone an effective treatment for cancer. It can be a valuable tool, however, for cancer prevention and treatment.

Cancer Lifeline hopes this book assists you in making choices that feel right for you. Happy reading and healthy eating!

CANCER LIFELINE
WE HELP PEOPLE LIVE WITH IT

Cancer Lifeline is a 24-hour support system—a lifeline—for people living with cancer. Our Lifeline volunteers are professionally trained and know how to listen, what to say, and when to offer help. They care.

Cancer Lifeline was founded by Gloria Gutkowski, who was diagnosed with breast cancer in 1970. It didn't take long for Gloria to see the void in services provided to cancer patients and their families and friends. Even though she had supportive family and friends, there was no one to help her understand the disease or empower her to make decisions that were right for her, no one to talk with about her feelings, fears, and concerns.

Gloria started talking to doctors, nurses, and social services providers, assessing the need for emotional support, information, and resources for people coping with the cancer experience. The response was very positive and, as a result, Cancer Lifeline was born in the summer of 1973.

During its first year, Cancer Lifeline qualified for United Way funding, and 20 volunteers were trained to provide counseling and resource referral via telephone. By the end of 1974, 250 calls had been received; in 1980 the organization served more than 1,500 people; and in 1990 that number jumped to 4,000. In 1994, 30 direct service volunteers gave 8,432 hours of their time to Cancer Lifeline and provided support to 4,500 people.

Over the years, Cancer Lifeline callers have expressed a variety of needs. They want reasons to hope, caring support, a chance to make their own decisions, help talking with their families or doctors, ways to take control of their lives, and classes to give them new ways to manage.

We have developed numerous programs designed to meet the challenges encountered during the cancer experience. To meet our clients' needs, we offer, free of charge, the 24-hour Lifeline, our Family Support Program, Kids' Groups, and more.

Workshops and classes are offered regularly during the year. Movement Awareness, Relaxation and Stress Management, and Managing Cancer Pain classes serve the needs of both cancer patients and their families.

Cancer Lifeline has published *What to Eat Now* in an effort to empower cancer patients, caregivers, and others to participate actively in creating a healthful nutrition plan.

"Throughout the last two decades, Cancer Lifeline has been helping cancer patients and those who care about them find ways to bring choice and control back into their lives," says Barbara Frederick, Cancer Lifeline's executive director. "Although cancer may impair a person's health, it doesn't need to take away one's dignity or ability to guide their own life."

MAKING HEALTHIER FOOD CHOICES

Many in the scientific community believe that 30 percent of all cancers are related in some way to what we eat. Some foods may *cause* cancer, some foods may *promote* cancer, and some foods may *protect* against cancer. For the person with cancer, a healthy diet has been shown to make a crucial difference in enhancing the overall recovery process.

By reshaping your diet—to *include* foods that may protect against cancer and *avoid* foods that may promote cancer—you can become an active participant in fighting disease, speeding your recovery, and improving your sense of well-being. We hope the following information will give you the details and tips you need to accomplish these goals—and have some fun in the process.

The Top 10 "Super Foods"

Although there are many nourishing foods, a number of "super foods" have been singled out as possibly protecting against disease and promoting good health. Adding these foods to your diet as often as possible is a great step toward better health, whether you're a cancer patient or just a person who's committed to living a healthier life. Nutritionist Rachel Keim has selected 10 favorites. Throughout this section you'll find tips for putting them to good use, and many of our recipes include these items as ingredients.

Here are our Top 10 "Super Foods"

1. Cruciferous vegetables
2. Garlic
3. Carotenoid-rich foods
4. Yogurt
5. Beans
6. Soybeans
7. Citrus fruit
8. Fiber-rich foods
9. Fish
10. Mushrooms

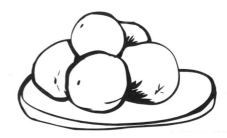

1. Cruciferous Vegetables

Possible Benefits

Some of the first foods linked to cancer protection were the *cruciferous vegetables:* broccoli, brussels sprouts, cabbage (red, white, napa and savoy), cauliflower, kale, Swiss chard, parsnips, watercress, radishes, bok choy, collard greens, kohlrabi, rutabaga, turnips, and mustard greens.

In a University of Minnesota study in the 1970s, a group of animals fed a diet rich in cruciferous vegetables had a significantly lower rate of cancer compared with a group of similar animals not fed cruciferous vegetables. Since then, two *phytochemicals* (substances found in plants) in cruciferous vegetables, *indoles* and *sulphoraphane*, have been identified as possibly being protective against cancer in humans. Cruciferous vegetables are also rich in fiber, vitamin C, and selenium—all of which may provide protection against cancer.

Optimizing Cruciferous Vegetables

"The fresher the better" is a good approach when choosing cruciferous vegetables. Select organically grown vegetables if they're available. They taste better and greatly reduce the risk of ingesting harmful chemicals.

It's best to eat cruciferous vegetables either raw or lightly cooked—stop cooking while they're still a little crunchy. If you have to eat softer foods because of side effects related to treatment, cook the vegetables as much as you like. It's better to eat them soft than not to eat them at all.

Add cruciferous vegetables to salads, eat them raw with dips, steam them with a little lemon juice, or sauté in garlic and chicken broth. Experiment with adding them to soups, casseroles, and sauces.

2. GARLIC

Possible Benefits

Garlic has been used as a folk remedy throughout the world for thousands of years. Egyptian medical records reveal that garlic was used as a medicine as early as 1550 B.C.; the Chinese have been using it for more than 3,000 years; and Hippocrates, the Greek "Father of Medicine," prescribed eating garlic as a treatment for uterine tumors around 350 B.C.

In modern times, animal and laboratory experiments have shown that various compounds in garlic may be deadly to invading tumors but harmless to normal, healthy body cells. These compounds may also be effective at fighting bacterial infection and enhancing the immune system.

The National Cancer Institute, the United States Department of Agriculture, and Loma Linda University are studying garlic as an immune system enhancer, a cancer-preventive agent, a blood clot inhibitor, and an agent to lower high blood pressure. Sulfur compounds from garlic may inhibit both carcinogens and the enzymes that allow cancers to spread.

The white blood cells of people who eat garlic seem to be more effective at destroying cancer cells than the white blood cells of people who don't eat garlic. In fact, there is evidence that the incidence of certain cancers is lowest in areas of the world where garlic consumption is the highest.

Optimizing Garlic

Cutting or crushing a clove of garlic releases allicin, the antibacterial and antiviral compound in garlic. Because allicin is destroyed by heat, garlic needs to be ingested raw to serve as an antiviral remedy. Make a habit of adding it to salad dressings or dips. When you feel a cold coming on, try swallowing some diced garlic mixed with applesauce.

Many of the other beneficial compounds in garlic are not affected by heat, so you may also use it liberally when you cook. You'll reap the benefits of its healing properties *and* enjoy its wonderful flavor.

3. CAROTENOID-RICH FOODS

Possible Benefits

The National Cancer Institute recommends eating at least two servings of fruits and three of vegetables every day—and for good reason. While all produce is good for you, a number of fruits and vegetables may provide a protective effect against certain cancer-causing agents.

Deep green, yellow, orange, and red fruits and vegetables (like spinach, sweet potatoes, carrots, squash, bell peppers, cantaloup, mangoes, strawberries, nectarines, papayas, and apricots) are rich in nutrients and contain *carotenoids,* the best known of which is beta-carotene. Carotenoids contain *antioxidants* that may stimulate the immune system and protect cells against the oxidative damage linked to cancers.

Antioxidants are important in fighting *free radicals,* the by-products of the natural activity of oxygen in cells. Free radicals are very reactive and roam the body, damaging cells and the genetic material within them. This can hinder the natural ability of cells to resist the development of cancer.

Our cells have well-developed systems for fighting free radicals and mending the damage they cause by using antioxidants the cells manufacture themselves. We can assist the cells by *adding* antioxidants through the foods we eat. Many studies have reported a relationship between low risk for cancer and high consumption of foods containing antioxidants.

Carotenoids appear to work in several other ways as well. They may enhance communication among healthy cells and help to keep cancer cells from "running amok." Additionally, beta-carotene is transformed into retinoic acid, a substance which, some researchers say, can turn on and off genes that may play a role in cancer development.

Optimizing Carotenoids

When choosing carotenoids, the rule is "the darker the better." Selecting the darkest leafy vegetables and a rainbow of brightly colored fruits and vegetables will guarantee that you're adding a host of vitamins and minerals—and there's a good chance you're getting some cancer-inhibiting substances as well.

Eat any of the carotenoid-rich foods as often as you like. Many fresh fruits and vegetables can be washed, cut up, and stored in airtight containers so you'll have plenty of fresh, healthy foods readily accessible for snacks or cooking.

4. YOGURT

Possible Benefits

Fermented foods have long been important to most of the world's populations for their nutritional and therapeutic benefits. Yogurt is fermented milk.

Some animal and laboratory studies have shown that yogurt has antibacterial, antiviral, and antifungal effects. Lactobacillus, one of the active cultures found in yogurt, appears to stimulate the body's immune system by increasing the production of natural killer cells and interferon. Our immune system uses both the natural killer cells and interferon as weapons against tumor cells that invade the body.

The National Cancer Institute has determined that some malignant tumors shrink in patients who consume a steady diet of yogurt. Studies show that yogurt is especially effective against vaginal cancer.

Yogurt also provides important nutrients such as vitamins B6, B12, niacin, folic acid, and potassium, and increases the digestibility of lactose and protein.

Optimizing Yogurt

When buying yogurt, make sure the label lists "live" or "active" cultures; *Lactobacillus acidophilus* is especially desirable. Avoid yogurt with sugars or sugar substitutes. There are plenty of good nonfat or low-fat yogurts from which to choose.

Yogurt makes a tasty, healthy addition to salad dressings and dips, or it can be used as toppings for soups or potatoes. When you're baking, try yogurt as a substitute for part of the fat. And don't miss our recipe for Yogurt Protein Shake.

You can easily make a slightly more firm and less bitter yogurt, sometimes referred to as "yogurt cheese." Simply line a colander or strainer with cheesecloth and drain the yogurt over a bowl for a couple of hours or overnight in the refrigerator. If you must avoid milk products, try taking bacterial cultures directly in the form of lactobacillus supplements sold in most natural food stores and supermarkets.

5. BEANS

Possible Benefits

There are no two ways about it: beans (kidney, navy, black, white, red, pinto, lima, split peas, garbanzo, and lentils) are just an all-around great food. Most importantly for cancer survivors, beans contain several compounds that may have anti-cancer properties.

Protease inhibitors may retard the growth of human colon- and breast-cancer cells.

Isoflavones block the entry of estrogen into cells, which may reduce the risk of breast and ovarian cancer. It has also been found that beans may destroy certain cancer gene enzymes that can transform a normal cell into a cancer cell.

Phytosterols slow the reproduction of cells in the large intestine, which may slow the growth of some tumors.

Saponins are thought to interfere with the process by which DNA reproduces, and may prevent cancer cells from multiplying.

Beans are high in protein, carbohydrates, and fiber, but low in fat. What's more, they are an excellent source of B vitamins, calcium, potassium, zinc, and iron. Because beans are digested and released into the bloodstream gradually, they cause less fluctuation in blood sugar than most foods, which helps to minimize fatigue.

Optimizing Beans

Beans make wonderful, inexpensive additions to soups, salads, stews, pasta, and casseroles. They can also be used in dips and spreads. Have fun experimenting with seasonings and mixing different kinds of beans together. Be adventurous!

You'll want to introduce beans into your diet gradually so your digestive tract has a chance to adjust. The average person can start out by eating half a cup of beans every two or three days, then gradually work up to a cup or more per day.

6. SOYBEANS

Possible Benefits

Some scientists believe that differences in soy consumption explain why the incidence of breast cancer in Asian women is five to eight times lower than in American women, as well as why prostate cancer is lower in Asian men. Soybeans contain *phytoestrogens* (*phyto* means plant), natural substances chemically similar to the drug Tamoxifen. Researchers speculate that the phytoestrogens in soy may provide an antiestrogenic effect, blocking the cancer-promoting action estrogen is capable of having in breast tissue. In men, phytoestrogens seem to block testosterone, a male hormone that can spur the growth of prostate tumors.

Tofu, which is made from soybeans, contains the phytochemical *genistein,* which may interfere with the formation of new and rapidly developing blood vessels. Because tumors need a great deal of blood to survive, some researchers believe soy may help protect the body by starving the tumor of its blood supply and preventing the spread of cancer.

Soybeans also contain protease inhibitors, which some studies show may inhibit the development of colon, lung, mouth, liver, and esophageal cancers in animals.

And finally, *isoflavins*—which are prominent in soybeans and foods made from them—may act as antioxidants, carcinogen blockers, or tumor suppressors.

But what about the fat?

When you start to read the labels on tofu packages, you may be surprised by the percentage of fat contained in tofu. Yes, you're right, there *is* fat in tofu—it comes from the soybean oil. But tofu also contains protein, carbohydrates, fiber, and calcium. And you can choose low-fat varieties.

Optimizing Soy

Add the silken, firm-style tofu to any stir-fry, a casserole, or a pot of spicy chili, and it soaks up the flavors of the other ingredients. Sauté it with garlic, red pepper, ginger, and soy sauce for a delicious main dish. Blend silken, soft-style tofu into shakes, salad dressings, or dips. The silken tofu in the cardboard container has a long shelf life, so you can always keep some on hand. Tofu omelets with lots of vegetables are also terrific. Other good soybean products include soy milk, tempeh, and miso.

Soy products are now available in everything from chocolate soy milk to soy-based meat substitutes that resemble turkey, chicken, hamburger, or bologna. Be cautious, however, because many of these products are high in fat. Be sure to read labels and make the lowest-fat choices.

7. CITRUS FRUIT

Possible Benefits

Citrus fruit is packed with the cancer-inhibiting substances vitamin C, flavonoids, limonenes, and terpenes. Cells in the immune system, including T cells and phagocytes, need vitamin C and flavonoids to function properly. Both are antioxidants, which block access of carcinogens to cells and/or suppress malignant changes in cells. Flavonoids may also hamper the ability of hormones to bind to cells and as a result may inhibit cancer development.

Studies conducted both in laboratories and with human subjects show that vitamin C helps prevent the formation of *nitrosamines*, potent carcinogens formed during digestion of nitrites, preservatives found in processed meats such as hot dogs, bacon, ham, and sausage. Vitamin C is also essential for healthy gums, teeth, bones, body cells, and blood vessels.

Limonene is a phytochemical found in citrus fruits that accelerates the enzyme production that may help dispose of potential carcinogens.

Terpenes are believed to increase those enzymes known to break down carcinogens and decrease cholesterol.

Citrus fruit is also a good source of fiber. What's more, lemons and pineapple may stimulate the liver and help it process toxins.

Optimizing Citrus

Oranges, grapefruit, tangerines, pineapple, lemons, and limes are all excellent choices. Eat them as often as you like. The fruit itself is the best choice because of the benefits of the fiber, but citrus juice is good, too. If you have mouth or throat sores, avoid citrus fruits until the sores heal.

8. FIBER-RICH FOODS

Possible Benefits

Dietary fiber is material from plant cells that humans cannot digest or can only partially digest. It prevents constipation and helps move food, along with potential cancer-causing substances, through the intestines and out of the body. Fiber is found in whole grains, fruits, beans and vegetables. Its protective effect is widely supported by both human and animal studies.

Dietary fiber consumption is associated with a low risk of developing colon cancer. Studies in 1960 of the Bantu tribe of rural South Africa revealed a very low incidence of colon cancer. Tribal members also excreted large quantities of feces, which was related to the large volume of fiber they consumed.

Fiber acts to speed the passage of food through the gastrointestinal tract and to eliminate harmful substances from the body. The refining processes in developed countries have removed the fiber from grain and other foods. Researchers theorize this fiber loss is connected to the higher incidence of diseases that include cancer of the colon and rectum.

There also may be links between constipation, fiber intake, and breast cancer. One study found that women who had two or fewer bowel movements per week had 4.5 times the risk of precancerous breast changes as women who had a bowel movement more than once a day. A Dutch study which evaluated women on the basis of grain intake found that women who ate the most grain had less than half the risk of developing breast cancer of women who ate less grain. It has been shown that fiber may have a cancer-preventing effect on estrogen, a hormone linked to breast cancer.

Optimizing Fiber

You can easily get more fiber in your diet by beginning to make some simple changes in the way you eat. Try bran cereals, fresh or dried fruit instead of fruit juice, brown rice instead of white rice, whole-wheat bread in place of white bread, and beans instead of meat. It will probably take your body a little time to get used to extra fiber, so start out with just a few additions, then gradually add a few more every week.

Eat more beans, fruits, and vegetables. Have some fun changing the flavor and texture of your home-baked cookies, muffins, and breads by adding small amounts of different grains. Oats, rye, millet, corn, and buckwheat are good choices because they are whole grains with no fiber removed. For breakfast, add whole grains to your diet in the form of hot or cold cereals such as oatmeal and polenta.

9. FISH

Possible Benefits

Fish is rich in protein, iron, B vitamins, and other nutrients, and can take the place of meats that are high in saturated fat. Fish oil is known for its beneficial effects against the damage caused by heart disease. Some studies show fish oil may prevent the development and growth of colon and breast cancer.

Researchers investigated why natives of Greenland, who eat a diet very high in fat, have a low death rate from heart disease. The results pointed to the abundance of fish in the native diet, the oils in those fish, and the omega-3 fatty acids contained in those oils.

Omega-3 fatty acids found in some fish seem to play a significant role in the structure and function of body cells and systems. They and their hormone-like derivatives may help regulate the immune response, the inflammation response to injury
or infection, the formation of blood clots, blood pressure,
blood lipid levels, and many other body functions. They also
become part of the structure of cell membranes. Numerous
studies have shown that omega-3 fatty acids may also reduce
cholesterol, hypertension, heart disease, and the risk for developing breast cancer, rheumatoid arthritis, and multiple
sclerosis.

It has been shown that fish oil may interfere with the production of a hormone-like substance called *prostaglandin E2
(PGE2).* Breast cancer patients often produce too much PGE2,
which hinders their immune system's ability to fight cancer
cells.

Optimizing Fish

Make a habit of eating fish frequently, either poached, baked,
or lightly sautéed with some garlic. Excellent choices include
lentinan water-packed white albacore tuna, trout, salmon, herring, sardines, mackerel—all particularly good sources of
omega-3 fatty acids. These "fat fish" store fat in their muscles,
the part of the fish we eat. In contrast, lean fish (white fish
such as cod) store fat in their livers, and people generally don't
eat fish livers.

10. MUSHROOMS

Possible Benefits

Mushrooms have been revered in Asia as potent medicines for
thousands of years. In fact, Chinese emperors and Japanese
royalty drank mushroom teas and concoctions to achieve vital-
ity and long life.

At the very least, mushrooms are tasty, fun to cook, and nutritious. They contain some protein and a variety of vitamins and minerals. There is evidence that shiitake, maitake, and reishi varieties also contain *polysaccharides,* substances that may enhance the immune system and provide anticancer protection.

Some researchers believe polysaccharides may activate *macrophages*, a type of white blood cell which filters the blood and destroys cancer cells, viruses, and bacteria. Macrophages also signal other white blood cells to seek out and destroy cancer cells. One study of maitake mushrooms showed that an extract of this mushroom completely eliminated tumors in 40 percent of the animals tested, while 90 percent of the tumors were eliminated in the remaining 60 percent of the animals.

The shiitake contains *lentinan*, an antiviral substance that may stimulate the immune system to produce more interferon, a natural compound known to fight cancer and viruses.

Studies on the protective qualities of the shiitake, maitake, and reishi mushrooms have only been done using mushroom extract, so it isn't known whether eating fresh mushrooms in relatively small quantities will provide any protective effects. Nevertheless, mushrooms are a healthy, nutritious food that may have medicinal properties, so feel free to consume them liberally.

Optimizing Mushrooms

Use shiitake, maitake, or reishi mushrooms in place of some or all of more common mushrooms such as button mushrooms. They make tasty additions to casseroles and soups, stir-fries, and salads, and can be added to gourmet or everyday recipes.

Shiitake and button mushrooms are readily available in many grocery stores. Locating maitakes and reishis may be more challenging; start the search at Asian grocery stores.

✓ Honorable Mentions

Our Top 10 is not a comprehensive listing of the foods that may provide protection against cancer. Others include:

1. ▲ Tomatoes
2. ▲ Green tea
3. ▲ Cucumbers
4. ▲ Grapes
5. ▲ Onions
6. ▲ Radishes
7. ▲ Parsley
8. ▲ Chile peppers
9. ▲ Asparagus

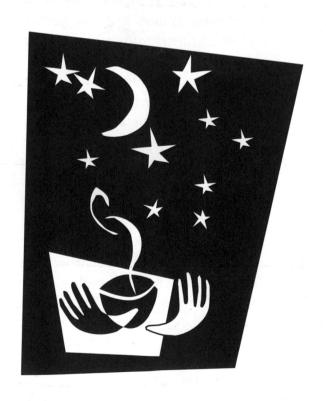

NUTRIENTS THAT PROMOTE GOOD HEALTH

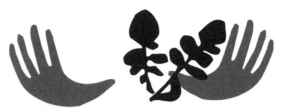

Getting all the nutrients you need in order to run your body efficiently is important for everyone, but it's especially important for cancer survivors. As your body is recovering from disease, it needs all the help it can get to repair and rebuild healthy tissue. Because eating may be more difficult during recovery, it is advantageous to pack as many nutrients as possible into the foods you *do* eat.

Your body requires six basic nutrients. Water is the nutrient needed in the greatest quantity, followed by protein, carbohydrates, fat, vitamins, and minerals. Protein, carbohydrates, and fat are called *macronutrients* because your body needs them in large quantities. Vitamins and minerals are called *micronutrients* because your body needs them in smaller amounts.

WATER

You may not think of water as one of the key nutrients, but it is. Water makes up approximately 50 to 60 percent of the body's weight. It brings to your body's cells the exact nutrients they need and carries away waste products. Water helps your body digest food, transport nutrients, maintain normal body temperature, flush toxins, and remove waste products.

It is typically recommended that you drink six to eight glasses of water throughout the day. However, you may need more if you're on chemotherapy, or less if your sodium level is out of balance. Your nutritionist, nurse, or doctor can advise you on the amount right for you.

Plain water is best, but you can also drink mineral waters (choose varieties without sodium added), bottled water flavored with fruit essence, or fruit juice diluted with sparkling water. Herbal tea, without caffeine, is also a good choice. Many people like to keep a bottle of water with them at all times to make drinking more convenient.

Limit your consumption of caffeinated sodas, coffee, and alcohol. When you *do* drink these beverages, don't count them as part of your daily fluid intake. They have a *dehydrating* effect and actually rob your body of fluid.

MACRONUTRIENTS

The macronutrients—protein, fat, and carbohydrates—are the body's primary source of fuel, and play a major role in maintaining the balance of many of the hormones and enzymes in the body. Two of those hormones, insulin and glucagon, control the sugar levels in the blood and enzymes that balance the body's metabolic processes. These processes help to regulate the immune response, the formation of blood clots, the inflammation response to injury or infection, and many other body functions.

A diet that provides a healthy balance of macronutrients is especially important if your body has been stressed or compromised by disease and treatment.

Protein—The Body's Building Blocks
Protein is used by the body to build, maintain, and repair tissue. It helps regulate many of the body's chemical processes. The "average" male needs approximately 54 grams of protein

a day and the "average" female needs about 45 grams per day. However, during cancer treatment your body is under a great deal of stress and you may need more protein than usual to repair and rebuild tissue.

How much protein do you need? Need for protein varies from person to person. Your need will probably fluctuate as you progress through treatment and recovery. Use this formula to find out how much protein you need during treatment, and ask your nurse, doctor, or nutritionist for additional guidelines.

Your normal body weight_____ pounds

Your desired weight_____ pounds

Your minimum daily protein requirement = desired weight (in pounds) x 0.5_____ grams of protein per day

If you are losing weight, increase your protein intake to:

Desired weight x 0.7_____ grams of protein per day

2 Protein Sources

There are proteins in most foods we eat, but some foods have more than others. Here are a few examples.

About 7 grams of protein:
    1 ounce lean meat, poultry, fish
    ½ cup legumes
    ¼ cup tofu
    1 cup broccoli or brussels sprouts
    ½ cup cottage cheese
    1 cup egg noodles
    7 ounces milk or yogurt
    1 ounce cheese
    2 tablespoons peanut butter
    1 to 2 ounces nuts or seeds

About 3 grams of protein:
    1/3 cup cooked rice
    1/2 cup cooked cereals and grains
    1 slice of bread

About 2 grams of protein:
    1 cup raw vegetables
    1/2 cup cooked vegetables

An important consideration when choosing protein is: *how easy is it to digest?* Red meat, for example, may not be the best choice because it moves slowly through the stomach and intestines, exposing the walls of the colon to cancer-causing substances for larger periods of time.

Complete and Incomplete Proteins

A *complete protein* contains all eight of those amino acids your body needs but can't produce on its own. All animal proteins are complete proteins.

Incomplete proteins contain different combinations of the eight amino acids, but not all of them. All plant proteins are incomplete proteins. However, soy is the most complete of all the plant proteins.

While animal products are a source of complete protein, most are high in saturated fat and contain a limited variety of other nutrients. Therefore, it's advisable to use meat as one source of protein, but not the *only* source. Good choices of animal protein include skinless chicken and turkey; fish and shellfish; lean cuts of red meat (round, loin, or flank); low-fat and nonfat cheeses; and other nonfat dairy products such as yogurt and milk. Avoid processed meats, organ meats, and fatty cuts of red meat.

By combining legumes, grains, nuts, seeds, and vegetables in your diet, you can create complete protein that offers greater amounts and wider varieties of vitamins and minerals and less

NUTRIENTS THAT PROMOTE GOOD HEALTH

saturated fat than animal protein. Excellent sources of plant protein include tofu and other soy products, dried beans, brown rice, barley, and nuts such as almonds and walnuts.

Legumes are the fruit or seeds of leguminous plants such as kidney beans, soybeans, split peas, lentils, black-eyed peas, and lima beans. Their specially adapted root systems trap nitrogen in the soil and turn it into compounds that become part of the seed. The result? Legumes are richer in high-quality protein than most plant foods.

Remember that you don't have to combine these foods in the same meal—just eat a well-rounded selection of them through-out the day. Some complete-protein combinations you may want to try include:

▲ Beans and rice
▲ Beans and tortillas
▲ Bread and peanut butter
▲ Tofu and vegetables
▲ Bean and vegetable soup

Creating Complete Plant Protein

Combine foods from any two of the following columns to create a complete protein.

Legumes	Grains	Nuts & Seeds	Vegetables
Dried lentils	Rice	Cashews	Broccoli
Soy products such as tofu	Whole grain bread	Sesame seeds	Leafy greens
Dried peas	Barley	Almonds	Zucchini
Dried beans	Bulgur	Walnuts	Sweet potatoes
Peanuts	Oats	Nut butters	
	Cornmeal	Other nuts	
	Pasta		

If you read the information about creating complete proteins and your first reaction was "Great! I can eat all the peanut butter sandwiches and cashews I want!"—don't rush to the store quite yet. Yes, these food combinations contain complete protein, but they also contain loads of fat. As a guideline, eating 10 walnuts or almonds a day gives you a great boost of protein and minerals. Just don't overdo it!

Carbohydrates—The Body's "Preferred Fuel"

Carbohydrates are the body's primary source of immediate fuel. They offer a wide variety of nutrients that nourish the brain and central nervous system, provide energy, and help keep your bowel movements regular. Fiber found in complex carbohydrates stimulates the muscles of the digestive tract so they retain their health and tone. This in turn speeds up the transit time of materials—including those linked with cancer—through the colon. Fiber also maintains bowel health and may reduce the incidence of colon cancer.

Complex and Simple Carbohydrates

Complex carbohydrates are whole foods that contain all their fiber and vitamins, unlike simple carbohydrates, which have had their fiber and vitamins removed. Complex carbohydrates have many components, so it takes time for them to be broken down and reach your bloodstream. They make the best all-around fuel because they "burn" slowly and can help increase your feelings of stamina.

Simple carbohydrates, on the other hand, are digested and absorbed into the bloodstream more quickly. They don't provide the feelings of stamina and endurance that complex carbohydrates do. They promote greater increases in blood sugar and insulin levels, which can lead to increased fatigue.

Carbohydrate Sources

Complex carbohydrates that are healthy choices include dried beans and peas, whole-grain breads and cereal, oatmeal, polenta, brown rice, vegetables, and whole-grain pastas.

Limit your use of simple carbohydrates such as processed baked goods containing lots of sugar, sweetened cereals made from white flour rather than whole grains, candy, and soda pop. Try to use less white rice and pastas made from white flours.

Fat—A Little Goes a Long Way

The body is constantly using small amounts of fat for fuel. While some fat is essential for good health, most people consume too much of it. Cancers of the breast, prostate, and colon, as well as obesity and an increased risk of heart attack, are all linked to high fat consumption.

A widely publicized 1992 study reported that there is no link between fat and breast cancer, but *decades of research* indicate that there really is such a connection. In fact, most studies of human populations suggest an association between dietary fat and breast cancer, a link further supported by animal studies.

While excess fat doesn't *cause* cancers, it may promote and speed the development of cancer by:

▲ Causing the body to secrete more of certain hormones, including estrogen, that create an environment that is favorable to cancer development.

▲ Promoting the secretion of bile into the intestine. (It is thought that bile is then converted by organisms in the colon into compounds that cause cancer.)

▲ Becoming incorporated into cell membranes and changing

them so that they lack the defenses they need to block entry of carcinogenic substances.

▲ Decreasing the function of certain components of the immune system.

Population studies around the world show that people who get 20 percent or less of their total calories from fat have fewer diseases and health problems, including cancers, heart attacks, and strokes. By contrast, the typical American diet includes almost 40 percent fat! Many experts believe that amount should be reduced to no more than 30 percent, and preferably to 20 percent.

Finally, it has been shown that a low-fat diet may enhance the successful outcome of cancer therapy. In both animals and humans, a low-fat diet seems to improve cell membrane fluidity, which can allow for better oxygen supply to tissue and may lessen the symptoms of chemo- and radiation therapies.

Types of Fat

Saturated fat comes from tropical oils such as coconut milk and palm oil, and animal sources such as butter, meat, lard, and whole-milk products. Saturated fat is usually solid at room temperature. It is linked with heart disease and cancer.

Polyunsaturated fat comes from plant sources, such as corn and safflower oils, and is liquid at room temperature. It lowers both LDL ("bad" cholesterol) *and* HDL ("good" cholesterol). While better for you than saturated fat, polyunsaturated fat is still linked to cancers because of the total fat that adds up in the diet.

Omega-3 fatty acids—found in fish such as salmon and mackerel, as well as in leafy vegetables, flax seeds and flax oils— have an anticlotting action that may be effective in preventing heart attack and stroke. Population studies do not seem to link omega-3 and monounsaturated fats with promoting cancer. In fact omega-3 fats may even protect against the cancer-promoting effects of other forms of fat.

Monounsaturated fat comes from plant sources and includes olive, canola, peanut, sesame, avocado, and walnut oils. Nuts, and butters made from nuts, fall into this category. Monounsaturated fat, which is liquid at room temperature, reduces only the damaging LDL and leaves HDL untouched. People in Greece and Italy who consume lots of monounsaturated fat tend to have less incidence of heart disease and cancer, even though they have fairly high-fat diets. Research indicates that olive oil is the best choice for monounsaturated fat.

Hydrogenated fat (also called *trans fat*) is a polyunsaturated fat that has been chemically changed to create a spreadable product (one that is solid at room temperature), and is found in margarines and baked goods. In the transformation process, hydrogenated fat loses its unsaturated character and the health benefits that go with that.

Which Is Better—Butter or Margarine?
Neither! Butter is a saturated fat, margarine is a hydrogenated fat, and both are linked to heart disease and cancer. Olive oil is a better choice, or try our recipe for Better than Butter.

Desirable Fat Sources
If you're losing weight and are being encouraged to eat more calories in the form of fat, be sure to select fat that has nutrients in it. For example, choose:

▲ Milk shakes made with soy milk, yogurt, and/or tofu instead of with ice cream—see our Yogurt Protein Shakes recipes

▲ Peanut butter or almond butter, instead of butter, spread on bread or waffles

▲ Avocado instead of mayonnaise in a sandwich or on toast

▲ Fatty fish such as salmon instead of white fish or meat

To cut back on fat, begin choosing low-fat or nonfat milk products, lean broiled, baked, or braised meats, skinless fish or poultry, and fresh fruits and vegetables prepared without oils or cream. Try getting more of your protein from plant sources such as dried peas and beans, tofu, grains, and vegetables.

MICRONUTRIENTS

While your body needs micronutrients in smaller quantities than it does macronutrients, each of them is essential to achieving and maintaining good health.

Vitamins—Necessary for Life and Growth

Vitamins are chemical compounds the body requires in small amounts. While they don't provide energy, they help the body process and use the energy it gets from food. Most vitamins cannot be made by the body or are not made in sufficient quantities to meet the body's needs, so they must be supplied by food.

Diets rich in foods containing antioxidant vitamins—E, C, and beta-carotene (a plant form of vitamin A)—may protect against many forms of cancer, including oral, esophageal, and reproductive-system cancers. Diets low in vitamin A actually may increase risk for some cancers.

Nobel Prize–winning scientist Linus Pauling found that vitamin C works to strengthen the immune system and keep tumors from spreading, by migrating through the body to find and destroy stray cancer cells. Vitamin C, he reported, has remarkable powers for detoxifying toxic substances in the human body, including carcinogens.

Fruit and vegetable intake, and most notably vitamin C intake, have been found to provide a consistent protective effect against breast cancer. It is theorized that if women in North America increased their fruit and vegetable intake to reach an average 380 mg of vitamin C per day, the breast cancer risk in the population would be decreased by 16 percent.

Vitamins E, C, and Beta-Carotene Sources
Fruits: fruits and juices of citrus, apricots, kiwis, mangoes, peaches, strawberries, cantaloup and other melons, papayas
Vegetables: carrots, broccoli, brussels sprouts, sweet potatoes. red and green peppers, tomatoes, peas, spinach

Supplements to Your Diet
It's important to get as many of your daily nutrients as possible from vitamin-rich *whole foods,* such as fruits, vegetables, beans, and grains. This is because some substances contained in whole foods are not available in supplement form. In fact, there may be in foods important substances of which we aren't even aware.

Since optimal nutrition is essential when you're fighting disease, taking supplements may be a rational and beneficial choice. It is believed that good nutrition decreases recovery time, speeds return of the senses of smell and taste to normal, promotes wound healing, and helps restore a sense of well-being more quickly.

Talk to your doctor, nurse, or nutritionist before taking supplements if you're in treatment. Supplements may interfere with chemo- or radiation therapy.

Minerals—The Body's Regulators
Minerals are found in all body tissues and fluids. They help the body build tissue, regulate body processes, maintain fluid balance, and use the energy from food. They do not *provide* energy.

It is essential that we consume enough minerals to ensure the proper functioning of our bodies. For cancer survivors who may be eating less, it can be more difficult to get sufficient quantities of minerals, including potassium, magnesium, calcium, iron, and selenium.

Calcium may have some preventive value related to colon cancer. Malignancies may be more common in people who have reduced selenium levels in their blood, especially if their diet is also lacking in vitamins A and C. Selenium seems to promote antioxidant activities and may help prevent cancer.

Treatment and its side effects can result in deficiencies in essential minerals, so try to pack your diet with whole foods—fruits, vegetables, beans, grains—that can help your body replace them.

Mineral Sources

1. Calcium: green leafy vegetables such as spinach, bok choy, and kale; sardines or salmon; tofu made with calcium sulfate; broccoli; kidney beans; cabbage; whole-wheat bread; 1 percent or nonfat milk products; turnip greens; sea vegetables

2. Iron: beet greens or Swiss chard, green peas, spinach, dates, lima beans, Boston or Bibb lettuce, parsley, raisins, meat, egg yolks, whole grains, dried beans

3. Magnesium: spinach, sunflower seeds, lima beans, garbanzo beans, figs, potatoes, cashews, squash, broccoli

4. Potassium: potatoes, molasses, raisins, bananas, lima beans, cabbage, carrots, broccoli, cauliflower, mushrooms, squash, yams, sweet potatoes, avocados, salmon, tuna, peanut butter

5. Selenium: whole grains, seafood, brewer's or nutritional yeast

Sea Vegetables . . . A Great Source of Minerals

Sea vegetables such as kombu, hijiki, and wakame are excellent sources of calcium, magnesium, and potassium, and they add minerals without changing the flavor of foods.

For dishes that cook longer than an hour, toss in whole or cut-up sea vegetables at the beginning of the cooking period. For dishes that cook less than an hour, soak the vegetables for 10 minutes, until they're soft enough to cut, then cut them up and throw them in.

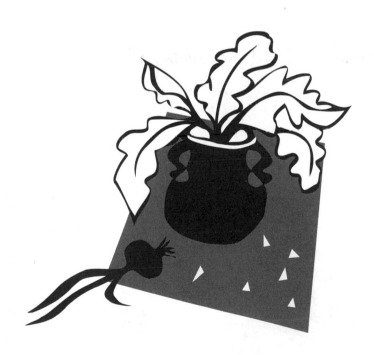

CREATING A HEALTHIER DIET

We have discussed the possible cancer-inhibiting properties of the Top 10 "Super Foods," as well as the importance of getting the "right" quantities of water, the macronutrients, and the micronutrients.

The next logical question is: "What exactly are *the right* quantities of all these components, and how do I begin to put them together for a healthier diet?"

6 Basic Food Groups

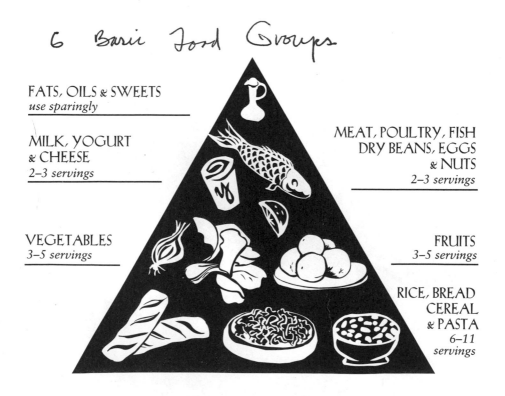

FATS, OILS & SWEETS
use sparingly

MILK, YOGURT
& CHEESE
2–3 servings

MEAT, POULTRY, FISH
DRY BEANS, EGGS
& NUTS
2–3 servings

VEGETABLES
3–5 servings

FRUITS
3–5 servings

RICE, BREAD
CEREAL
& PASTA
*6–11
servings*

The Food Pyramid—developed by the U.S. Department of Agriculture/U.S. Department of Health and Human Services—illustrates the six basic food groups and the daily amounts of various foods you should eat to get all the needed nutrients. Remember to:

▲ Select the bulk of your food from the lower levels of the pyramid, with emphasis on fruits, vegetables, and *whole* grains (whole-grain rice, pasta, and bread, rather than white).

▲ Choose milk products that are 1 percent milk fat or nonfat.

▲ Eat lots of beans. While beans are listed near the top of the pyramid, in the same group with animal products, they could be placed at the base of the pyramid. Beans are an excellent, nonfat source of carbohydrates, fiber, vitamins, and protein.

The Food Pyramid recommends two to three servings, three to five servings, etc. Which number is right for you? If your daily calorie intake is in the 1,600 range, eat the smaller number of servings per day. If it's closer to 3,000 per day, eat the larger number of servings.

What Counts as One Serving?

It may seem like eating all those servings of all those foods is practically impossible. But take a look at your daily intake and you may be surprised how close you are to meeting the daily requirements.

Eat any one item listed below and you have eaten the equivalent of one serving.

MILK, YOGURT, CHEESE (NONFAT OR LOW-FAT)
▲ 1 cup of milk or yogurt
▲ 1½ ounces of natural cheese
▲ 2 ounces of processed cheese

MEAT, POULTRY, FISH, DRIED BEANS, EGGS, NUTS
▲ 2 to 3 ounces of cooked lean meat, poultry, or fish
▲ ½ cup cooked dried beans, 1 egg, or 2 tablespoons of peanut butter count as 1 ounce of lean meat

VEGETABLES
▲ 1 cup raw leafy vegetables
▲ ½ cup of other vegetables (cooked or raw)
▲ ¾ cup vegetable juice

FRUIT
▲ 1 medium apple, banana, or orange
▲ ½ cup chopped, cooked, or canned fruit
▲ ¾ cup fruit juice

BREAD, CEREAL, RICE, PASTA
▲ 1 slice of bread
▲ 1 ounce ready-to-eat cereal
▲ ½ cup cooked cereal, rice, pasta

FATS, OILS, SWEETS
▲ No specific guidelines are given, but the message is clear: Use them sparingly.

Spending Your "Fat Budget"

If you're like most of us, you probably don't know how many grams of fat are in your favorite foods or how many grams of fat are appropriate to eat in a given day. The number of fat grams you should be eating is based on a percentage of the total calories you eat each day. That varies from person to person. If you've recently had chemotherapy, radiation, or surgery, your calorie needs may be higher than normal because body tissue is being repaired. Ask your doctor, nurse, or nutritionist to help you determine what caloric and fat intake is best for you.

Identifying Your Calorie Limit

▲ Underweight adults: multiply your body weight (in pounds) by 18.

▲ Normal-weight adults: multiply your body weight by 16.

▲ Overweight adults: multiply your body weight by 14.

You now have an estimation of the number of calories you need per day. For example, a 140-pound, underweight adult needs about 2,520 calories a day; a 140-pound, normal-weight adult needs about 2,240 calories a day; and an overweight, 140-pound adult needs about 1,960 calories a day. Some days you'll consume more calories, and some days you'll consume less. The idea is to *average* this number of calories.

Figuring Your Fat Limit

Now that you have an idea of your daily calorie requirement, check the following chart to see how many grams of fat you should be consuming. Choose whether you want to eat 20 percent, 25 percent or 30 percent of your total calories in fat. Remember, 30 percent is OK if you need to gain weight. Otherwise, 25 percent or 20 percent are great goals for maintaining a healthy weight and maximizing overall health.

As an example, let's say you need 2,000 calories per day and you want to keep your fat intake down to 20 percent of your daily calories. According to the chart, you'll want to strive to consume about 40 grams of fat per day.

Total daily calories	20% total calories	25% total calories	30% total calories
1,600 - 1,800	36 - 40 fat grams	44 - 50 fat grams	53 - 60 fat grams
1,800 - 2,000	40 - 44 fat grams	50 - 56 fat grams	60 - 67 fat grams
2,000 - 2,200	44 - 49 fat grams	56 - 61 fat grams	67 - 73 fat grams
2,200 - 2,400	49 - 53 fat grams	61 - 67 fat grams	73 - 80 fat grams
2,400 - 2,600	53 - 58 fat grams	67 - 72 fat grams	80 - 87 fat grams

Fat Limits Per Day

To find out how many fat grams are in your favorite foods and whether you're staying within your "fat budget," keep track of what you're eating for a while.

Buy a pocket-size "fat-gram counter" book. It will list the total fat, saturated fat, cholesterol, calories, fiber, and sodium in a wide variety of foods.

Record everything you eat, and add up the fat grams. After a few days, you'll probably have a pretty good idea where your "fat culprits" are lurking and where to begin cutting back if necessary.

You don't have to give up high-fat foods to see good results. Instead, try eating fewer fatty foods and making low-fat choices a little more often.

Protecting Yourself from Food-borne Illnesses

If you are living with a weakened immune system, your body is less effective in protecting you against illnesses carried by bacteria found in foods. Animal products in particular may contain harmful bacteria and other potentially dangerous pathogens. Remember, you cannot rely on your senses to determine if food is contaminated. Spoiled foods do not necessarily change in smell, taste, or appearance. Food can be unsafe to eat before it begins to smell.

The U.S. Department of Agriculture offers some suggestions to help you and your family lower the risk of food-borne illnesses when shopping, preparing, cooking, and storing dairy products and eggs, fresh meat, poultry, and seafood.

Check the "sell by" and "best used by" dates on the product. The further ahead the date is from the date you are shopping, the better. For fresh meat, poultry, and seafood, buy the item only if the date on the package is today's or yesterday's date.

Buy only refrigerated eggs and check for clean, uncracked shells. Store eggs in their original carton in the main section of the refrigerator.

Avoid raw eggs. Before using the eggs, make sure there are no visible cracks in the shell. When cooking with eggs make sure you cook them thoroughly. Sunny-side-up eggs are more likely to cause problems if harmful bacteria are present due to their short cooking time.

When you are in the store, buy eggs, milk, meats, fish, and frozen foods last.

Refrigerate or freeze meat, poultry, or fish as soon as you get home. Few food-borne bacteria can grow in the refrigerator, and none can grow in the freezer.

Cooking food thoroughly is the best protection you have against food-borne illness. Keep fresh meat, poultry, or fish away from other foods. Don't chop salad vegetables on a cutting board where you've just trimmed raw meat, poultry, or fish. Wash the cutting board, countertop utensils, and your hands with hot soapy water after contact with the fresh meats.

To prevent contamination, refrigerate leftovers within two hours after cooking or serving. Use the recommended storage times as a guide for keeping foods:

	In Refrigerator	In Freezer
Fresh meat	3-5 days	6-12 months
Hamburger	1-2 days	3-4 months
Fresh fish	1-2 days	2-3 months
Milk	5 days past carton date	1 month
Leftovers	1-2 days	2-3 months
Eggs	3-5 weeks	do not freeze in shell

MAKING FAVORITE RECIPES HEALTHIER

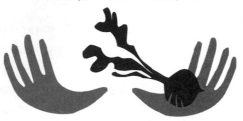

You can make your favorite recipes a little more nutritious with a few simple alterations.

LOWERING FAT CONTENT

▲ Cut the total fat in the recipe in half. For example, reduce ½ cup of olive oil to ¼ cup. Replace the fat with an equal amount of another liquid such as broth, water, wine, buttermilk, or yogurt. Try substituting applesauce, mashed bananas, or puréed prunes for fat if you're making something sweet.

▲ Whenever possible, use vegetable protein like beans, grains, legumes, and tofu instead of animal protein. Begin thinking of meat as a side dish rather than the main course.

▲ Start using leaner cuts of meat, or substitute skinless ground turkey or chicken breast. Try using fish in place of fatty meats.

▲ Substitute evaporated skim milk in recipes calling for cream, use nonfat or low-fat yogurt or sour cream instead of regular sour cream, and try skim or low-fat milk instead of whole milk. Low-fat or fat-free buttermilk is also available and can be purchased in powdered form.

▲ Remember that French-style breads have no fat, and some are available in whole-grain varieties.

▲ Experiment with nonfat dairy products and low-fat cheese.

▲ Try steaming, broiling, baking, grilling, or braising.

▲ Sauté foods in broth, water, or wine instead of oil, and use nonstick pans.

▲ Reduce the amounts of nuts and cheeses you use.

▲ Replace the shortening, butter, or margarine in recipes with our recipe for "Better than Butter."

▲ Substitute two egg whites for every egg called for. Eggs are a source of fat, but all the fat is in the yolk. Try nonfat egg substitutes.

LOWERING SUGAR & SALT CONTENT

Guidelines from the National Research Council state that Americans should eat no more than 10 percent of their total calories from sugar, and should keep their sodium intake to 2,000 mg or less a day. Sugar contains no nutrients—only calories. With that in mind, here are a few tips for decreasing the sugar and salt in your recipes.

Sugar
▲ Cut all sugar measurements in half.

▲ Experiment with alternative sweeteners. Familiar ones are applesauce, molasses, honey, and fruit juice concentrate. Less familiar ones include rice and barley sweeteners, Succanat, and date sugar. These can usually be found in the specialty section of a large supermarket or at a health food store. Note that because date sugar doesn't dissolve in liquid, it's not good in coffee, but it works well for baking.

▲ For every ¾ cup of liquid sweetener substituted for dry sweetener (honey instead of sugar, for example), decrease the amount of liquid in the recipe by ¼ cup or add an extra ¼ cup of flour.

▲ Frost cakes while still warm with a thin powdered sugar glaze rather than a thick layer of frosting.

Salt

▲ Eliminate salt or cut measurements in half.

▲ Skip or reduce the salt if the recipe calls for baking soda or baking powder; these items already contain sodium.

▲ Get creative with herbs and other seasonings rather than relying on salt. Season vegetables with lemon juice.

▲ Remember that all packaged spice mixes (taco, gravy, dressings, stew, spaghetti sauce, etc.) are extremely high in sodium. Make your own spice blends or purchase no-salt blends.

Seasoning Suggestions

Fruits:	Caraway, cinnamon, cloves, ginger, mint, parsley, tarragon
Vegetables:	Basil, caraway, chives, dill weed, marjoram, mint, nutmeg, oregano, paprika, rosemary, savory, tarragon, thyme
Salads:	Basil, chervil, chives, dill weed, marjoram, mint, oregano, parsley, tarragon, thyme
Rice:	Marjoram, parsley, tarragon, thyme, turmeric
Pasta:	Basil, fennel, garlic, paprika, parsley, sage
Seafood:	Chervil, dill weed, fennel, parsley, tarragon
Poultry:	Garlic, oregano, rosemary, sage, savory
Pork:	Coriander, cumin, ginger, sage, thyme
Lamb:	Garlic, marjoram, mint, oregano, rosemary, sage, savory
Beef:	Bay, chives, garlic, marjoram, savory

Increasing Fiber Content

▲ Choose whole-grain rather than refined flours. You can substitute whole wheat pastry flour for any or all of the white flour a recipe calls for. If you're incorporating other grains such as buckwheat, oats, or amaranth, do not substitute for more than a quarter of the total flour called for.

▲ Use brown rather than white rice, or try a mixture of half white and half brown. Experiment with other whole grains such as quinoa, millet, bulgur, or cornmeal, as suggested in our recipes.

▲ Try whole wheat or corn tortillas for burritos, casseroles, quesadillas, and nachos.

▲ Select a wide variety of fruits and vegetables, with emphasis on those in our list of Top 10 "Super Foods."

▲ Look for 100 percent whole wheat when buying bread or baked goods. (The word *whole* must come before the word *wheat* or you're not getting whole wheat. Don't be fooled.) Other grains—oats, corn, millet—do not have fiber removed when they are processed, so they don't need to have the word *whole* in front of their names on the label.

Secrets to Success

1. Change only one ingredient in a recipe at a time. That way, if your creation is less than a success, you'll know where the problem lies.

2. Start out slowly. You can always further reduce fat, sugar, and salt after your taste buds have adjusted.

3. Wait to announce the changes until you've served the dish and it has received rave reviews.

4. Accept progress without perfection. Every journey begins with the first step.

GETTING ORGANIZED

You and your family may have difficulty finding the time and energy to prepare healthy, nutritious snacks and meals, but eating right is ~~undoubtedly~~ more important now than ever before. The trick is to find ways to make shopping and food preparation as quick and easy as possible.

Here are some suggestions for stocking up on supplies you'll need for wholesome, healthy cooking and eating.

STOCKING UP

DRY STORAGE
Canned chicken broth, low-sodium
Vegetable broth, powder or canned low-sodium
Tuna, canned in water
Evaporated skim milk
Canned fruits in unsweetened juice
Canned tomatoes, low-sodium (purée, paste, sauce)
Canned beans, low-sodium varieties
Dried peas, beans, lentils
Nonstick olive or canola oil cooking spray
Whole grains—brown rice, bulgur, barley, millet, quinoa, polenta, oatmeal, bran
Popcorn (try low-fat microwave types)
Pasta, whole-grain varieties
Fresh garlic, potatoes, tomatoes, onions
Flour, white and whole wheat pastry
Baking soda and aluminum-free baking powder

Vinegars (balsamic, rice, red, white)
Low-sodium soy and Worcestershire sauces
A variety of dried herbs and spices and salt-free blends
Sun-dried tomatoes
Pure vanilla, peppermint, almond, and orange extracts

REFRIGERATOR STORAGE
Nonfat milk and yogurt
Low-fat cottage cheese, ricotta cheese, and cream cheese
Light or fat-free mayonnaise
Dijon mustard
Low-calorie or no-oil salad dressings
Fresh ginger and basil
Low-sugar jams and preserves
Extra virgin olive oil
Cold-pressed safflower or canola oil
Fruits, seasonal and locally grown, if possible
Vegetables, seasonal and locally grown, if possible
Corn and whole wheat tortillas
Fresh salsa
Peanut butter and/or almond butter

FREEZER STORAGE
Frozen unsweetened fruit juice concentrates
Frozen fruits
Frozen vegetables
Freshly grated Parmesan cheese
Shredded mozzarella, low-fat or part skim
Almonds and walnuts
Pumpkin, sesame, and sunflower seeds
Whole wheat bread crumbs
Whole grain breads, bagels, waffles
Flours (special grains such as spelt, buckwheat, amaranth)
Natural juice bars, sorbet, low-fat frozen yogurt

Handy Utensils, Equipment, and Books
Important

Sharp knives

Mixing bowls

Measuring cups and spoons

Steamer tray or basket

Nonstick skillet and bakeware

Salad spinner

Hand mixer

Blender

A few good low-fat cookbooks that list calorie and
fat contents for each recipe

Nice—But Not Essential

Rice cooker (also excellent for steaming vegetables)

Slow-cooker (Crockpot)

Food processor

Microwave oven

Popcorn popper

Egg separator

Hand blender

Knife sharpener

WEEKLY MEAL PLANNING

Sit down once a week with a low-fat cookbook or some of
your family's favorite recipes, modify them so they're lower in
fat and higher in nutrients, and plan a week's worth of dinners.
As you plan, keep your nutritional goals in mind. For example:
"I want to eat fish twice a week and beans twice a week. I
don't want to cook every night, so we'll go out one night, and
have leftovers at least once."

Create a shopping list that includes all the items you'll need for
the meals, plus any other items you've used up. Once again,
remember your nutritional goals: "We each need to eat at least

two servings of fruit a day and there are three of us, so we'll need 42 pieces of fruit for the week. We need to eat at least three servings of vegetables a day, so . . ."

By *planning ahead,* you can shop just once a week. (Planning also reduces your chances of resorting to processed, packaged, or fast foods when you're tired and hungry. These foods are often high in fat, salt, and sugar, and low in nutrients.)

Here is an example of a weekly dinner plan. The starred (*) recipes are included in this book.

Sunday
>   Quick White Bean Chili*
>   Green Salad
>   Corn Bread*

Monday
>   Braised Pork*
>   Brown Rice*
>   Minted Carrots
>   Chocolate Chip Mint Cookies* (bake extra and freeze
>   for later use)

Tuesday
>   Bean Burritos (fill tortillas with leftover pork and rice from
>   Monday, refried beans, and vegetables)
>   Steamed Cauliflower
>   Seasonal Fruit

Wednesday
>   Roasted Chicken*
>   Mashed Potatoes
>   Steamed Broccoli
>   Biscuits*

Thursday

Chicken Pita Pockets (sauté bite-size pieces of leftover chicken
with vegetables and fill pita pockets)
Seasonal Fruit
Chocolate Chip Cookies*

Friday

Eat out

Saturday

Salmon in Sun-Dried Tomato Sauce*
Steamed Greens
Polenta*

Save each week's meal plans in a notebook or file folder.
Favorite plans can be reused when you're short on time or
energy.

Don't expect to plunge right into writing weekly menus. For
starters, you could make a commitment to plan one week of
dinners this month. Next month, reuse the week of menus
you've made, and create one more. Soon you'll have lots of
weekly menus from which to draw.

MAKING GROCERY SHOPPING A BREEZE

Planning ahead may seem like more work, but when you know
what to look for, your grocery shopping gets easier. And you
come home with food you *like* that will also keep you healthy.

Getting the Most Out of Your Shopping Trips

▲ Keep a shopping list handy. Whenever you run out of something, jot it down. Keep the Top 10 "Super Foods" in mind as
you plan your shopping list.

▲ Go to the grocery store once a week with your list. Buy only
what's on the list.

▲ Get help from friends or family members.

▲ Shop at non-peak hours that fit your schedule.

▲ Don't shop when you're hungry. Opt for a healthy snack before going to the store.

Reading Food Labels Before You Buy

New, informative labels on most packaged foods can steer you away from fatty, sugary, or salty products and help you stock your cupboards with more nutritious foods instead. Important things to look for include:

▲ Serving size—if you're going to eat the equivalent of two servings, remember to double the figures listed for calories and nutrients;

▲ Calories, and calories that come from fat—compare these two numbers and you can figure out the approximate percentage of fat in the product;

▲ Total fat grams—this listing will help you decide if the product is within your "fat budget";

Nutrition Facts		
Serving Size 1 package		
Servings Per Container 1		
		Amount Per Serving
Calories 130 Calories from Fat 0		
		% Daily Value
Total Fat 0g		0%
Saturated Fat 0g		0%
Cholesterol 0mg		0%
Sodium 410 mg		17%
Total Carbohydrate 25g		9%
Dietary Fiber 2 g		7%
Sugars 3g		
Protein 4g		
Vitamin A 30% ● Vitamin C 60%		
Calcium 9% ● Iron 6%		

▲ Sodium content—a healthy amount of sodium to eat per day is from 2,000 to 3,000 mg.

You'll notice a column entitled "% Daily Value" on the new labels. It is designed to tell you how much of a day's worth of fat, carbohydrate, etc., the product contains. But there's a problem: The numbers are based on the "average" person who eats about 2,000 calories a day, with 30 percent of them coming from fat. Since caloric needs vary from person to person, and you are hopefully striving for a fat content less than 30 percent, these numbers are confusing. It's best to ignore them.

It pays to be wary of claims on product packages such as "95 percent fat-free." Hot dogs, luncheon meats, frozen meals, and ice cream packages, to name just a few, often make these claims, but BEWARE: these statements are probably referring to the fat percentage *by weight* rather than *by calories*.

Here's an example: If you eat two pats of butter, 100 percent of the calories are from fat. Drop two pats of butter in a glass of water, and you've made a beverage that is 96 percent fat-free. But drink it and you'll still swallow the two pats of butter. It doesn't matter to your body whether you eat the butter with or without the water. Either way, you get the *same amount of fat.*

You *can* trust these key words defined and regulated by the government:

▲ Fat-free: Less than 0.5 gram of fat per serving

▲ Low-fat: 3 grams of fat or less per serving (except for 2 percent low-fat milk, which has 5 grams per serving)

▲ Lean: Less than 10 grams of fat, 4 grams of saturated fat and 95 milligrams of cholesterol per serving

▲ Extra lean: Less than 5 grams of fat, 2 grams of saturated fat, and 95 milligrams of cholesterol per serving

▲ Very low sodium: 35 milligrams of sodium or less per serving

▲ Low sodium: 140 milligrams of sodium or less per serving

▲ High fiber: 5 grams of fiber or more per serving

▲ Good source of fiber: 2.5 to 4.9 grams of fiber per serving

Check the list of ingredients on the package. The most common food additives are sugar and salt, so watch the labels and limit products that include sugars and salt. Other terms indicating sugar are corn syrup, molasses, honey, fructose, sucrose, dextrose, and fruit juice concentrate. Other words for salt are sodium, sodium chloride, sodium bicarbonate, and monosodium glutamate.

For more information about reading food labels, contact your local American Heart Association or call 800-242-8721.

ONCE YOU'RE HOME FROM THE STORE

Doing these few chores as soon as you return from the grocery store will simplify snack and meal preparation for the rest of the week.

▲ Wash and dry the lettuce. Seal it in plastic containers or bags to keep it fresh.

▲ Wash and cut up vegetables as soon as possible, storing them in the same way as the lettuce so they're ready for easy use in lunches, snacks, stir-fries, casseroles, soups, and salads.

▲ Steam rice or soak beans for use in the next two or three days.

And remember, if you are the cancer patient or the caregiver, these are all things you can ask friends or family members to do when they ask the proverbial question, "Is there anything I can do to help?"

SIMPLIFYING MEAL PREPARATION

The next step is to make the cooking and cleanup process as effortless as possible.

▲ Store prepared lettuce, vegetables, and leftovers near the front of the refrigerator in a large see-through container or in baggies. Keep a list of the contents on the refrigerator door and a pencil nearby so you can cross off items when they've been eaten. This gives everyone in the house an instant reminder of what's available for quick snacks and meals, and what to put on the grocery list. It also encourages family members to be self-sufficient and fix foods themselves. These "ready to go" foods come in very handy when you're not feeling well enough to prepare meals.

▲ Stop by the salad bar at the grocery store or pick up ready-to-eat vegetables for a stir-fry if time or energy is limited.

▲ Chop or mince twice as much onion, garlic, or ginger as a recipe calls for and store the rest in a baggy in the freezer for later use.

▲ Grate cheese and carrots and peel potatoes on paper plates or towels to minimize cleanup.

▲ Use quick and healthy cooking techniques such as:
Poaching: Simmer foods in hot liquid just below the
    boiling point. No added fat is needed.
Steaming: Place foods in a steamer basket over boiling
    water. This helps foods retain their water-soluble vitamins.
Stir-frying: Cook small, uniformly sized pieces of food in a
    non stick wok or large skillet, using a small amount of oil,
    broth, wine, or water.

Microwaving: Put your microwave to use for defrosting, reheating, and steaming. Because minimal amounts of added fat or liquid are needed, microwaving reduces both the calories from added fat and the loss of water-soluble vitamins.

Slow-cooker (Crockpot) cooking.

Cooking more food than you need and freezing the left overs (label and date containers before freezing).

Choosing Fast Foods

When you don't have the time or energy to prepare meals from scratch, or at all, fast food may be your best available option. Here are some tips for selecting the healthiest fast food possible.

At fast-food restaurants:

▲ Choose restaurants that have low-fat selections. Many fast-food restaurants now have low-fat menu items.

▲ Select restaurants that provide a nutritional analysis of menu items. For example, Taco Time offers nutritional information showing how to order their entrées leaving off high-fat sauces. Check the amounts of fat, sodium, and sugar. Know what you're eating.

▲ Choose items listed as "Heart Healthy" on menus.

▲ Select the salad bar as an alternative to burgers and fries, but go easy on salad dressing, cheese, sunflower seeds, olives, bacon bits, and salads made with mayonnaise.

▲ Avoid fried items.

▲ Remove skin from chicken.

▲ Have the cook or sandwich maker hold all excess dressing, butter, tartar sauce, and mayonnaise from buns and meat.

▲ Order water, iced tea, diet soda, or nonfat milk instead of a shake or whole milk.

▲ Skip biscuits at breakfast time—they're usually loaded with fat. Fat-free muffins or bagels are good choices, or cereal with nonfat milk.

At the Grocery Store:

▲ Read labels carefully. Select entrées that contain 15 grams of fat or less, and no more than 500 to 800 mg of salt per serving. Try cutting back on products that list sugar as an ingredient.

▲ Look for low-fat products. Try different brands to see which ones you like best.

▲ Select foods made with soy or whole grains whenever possible.

QUICK MEAL IDEAS

✓ Breakfast

Hot or cold cereal
Vegetable omelet with garlic and mushrooms
Muesli with yogurt (check to make sure the yogurt has active cultures)
Breakfast burrito: scrambled eggs with beans and cheese wrapped in a whole-wheat tortilla
Tofu scramble: fresh tofu in sun-dried tomato sauce
Whole grain toast or French toast
Whole grain pancakes, muffins, or biscuits
Yogurt shakes: juice, yogurt, frozen berries, etc.

Lunch ✓

Egg or tuna salad sandwich made with nonfat plain yogurt and vegetables (try these in pita pockets)

Garden burgers

Canned soups

Baked potato topped with chopped vegetables, chili, or salsa

Rice and beans

Whole-grain pasta salads made with vegetables

Hummus with vegetables in pita bread

Dinner ✓

Tuna or chicken casserole with noodles or rice

Polenta

Stir-fry vegetables with tofu

Whole-grain pasta with pesto, clam sauce, or red sauce

Baked yams, sweet potatoes, or squash

Mashed potatoes (try adding a little garlic)

Rice cooked with lentils and kombu

COPING WITH POSSIBLE SIDE EFFECTS OF CANCER TREATMENT

Cancer, its treatment, and the worry and fear that accompany the whole experience may result in some side effects that make eating more difficult and food less appealing.

Side effects, and ways to overcome or minimize them, vary from person to person and potentially even during different phases of treatment and recovery. Some people don't experience any side effects, or just minor ones. Here we offer some possible solutions, and we recommend you just keep trying different approaches until you find the ones that work best for you.

It may be helpful to keep a little notebook with you at all times—in your purse or briefcase during the day, and beside your bed at night. Jot down notes about what seems to trigger side effects, remedies that work and don't work, and questions to ask your doctor, nurse, or nutritionist. Be sure to keep your doctor informed about the side effects you are experiencing. Books, support groups, and the Internet may give you opportunities to share tips and encouragement with other cancer survivors.

Good luck, and remember: Most side effects go away when the treatment comes to an end.

Managing Treatment-related Symptoms

Nausea

▲ Keep track of when you experience nausea, and its possible cause (time of day, foods, events, surroundings). Share this information with your caregivers.

▲ Ask your doctor or nurse about medicine to help control nausea.

▲ Talk to your nutritionist about ways to modify your diet to minimize symptoms.

▲ Ask family or friends to grocery shop and cook for you if the sight or smell of food nauseates you. Stay out of the kitchen, or even leave the house while meals are being prepared.

▲ Try cold foods, which tend to have less odor than hot foods.

▲ Eat what sounds good. Some people find that they need to avoid fatty, greasy, or fried foods; spicy, hot foods; foods with strong odors; and very sweet foods. Other people crave spicy foods and strong flavors.

▲ Choose foods such as:
   Angel food cake

Clear liquids
Frozen juice cubes
Fruits or vegetables that are soft or bland (canned peaches, mashed potatoes)
Oatmeal
Pretzels
Sherbet or sorbet
Skinned chicken (baked or broiled, not fried)
Toast and crackers
Yogurt

▲ Avoid your favorite foods when feeling nauseated—you may develop a permanent dislike for them if you link them with feeling sick.

▲ Eat small meals slowly and frequently, about every two or three hours.

▲ Rest, sitting up, for about an hour after meals.

▲ Drink or sip cold beverages throughout the day, except at mealtimes. Ginger and peppermint teas may be soothing, and they're good combined.

▲ Keep crackers beside your bed to nibble before getting up in the morning.

▲ If you're hospitalized, have the lids removed from your meals before the tray is brought into your room so most of the odors are dispersed in the hallway.

▲ Wear loose-fitting clothing.

▲ Breathe some fresh air, or try relaxation techniques such as meditation or listening to soothing music.

Recipe for Ginger Tea

1. Peel and chop a fresh, 1-inch piece of ginger root.

2. Boil it in about 3 cups of water for 20 minutes.

3. Cool and drink the liquid.

You may store the tea for a day, but it's best made fresh each day.

VOMITING

▲ Call your doctor if you feel nauseated. It's better to treat the problem *before* vomiting begins. Also call if vomiting continues longer than half an hour.

▲ Wait an hour after vomiting stops before eating or drinking.

▲ Drink small amounts of clear liquids beginning one hour after vomiting has stopped. A teaspoon every 10 minutes is a good place to start, then gradually increase to a tablespoon every 20 minutes, then 2 tablespoons every 30 minutes. Ginger Tea is a good choice.

▲ Begin with a liquid diet of teas and broths, then gradually work up to a soft diet of applesauce, mashed or sweet potatoes, well-cooked vegetables, oatmeal, and rice.

CONSTIPATION

▲ Drink 8 to 10 glasses of liquid every day. Try keeping a bottle of water with you at all times. Add lemon, orange, or lime to water to give it a refreshing flavor.

▲ Drink a warm beverage about half an hour before your usual time for a bowel movement. Try to drink it at about the same time every day to help your body establish a regular routine. Some people find that drinking warm lemon water or prune juice is helpful.

▲ Eat high-fiber foods such as raw fruits and vegetables, whole grains, nuts, prunes, and raisins. If you have trouble chewing raw fruits and vegetables, try grating or cooking them, skins and all.

▲ Add oat or wheat bran to foods such as casseroles and homemade breads. Consuming 2 tablespoons of wheat bran a day will make your stools softer and easier to pass. However, because bran absorbs water, make sure you drink at least eight glasses of water a day.

▲ Flaxseed oil, about 1 tablespoon a day, may be beneficial for constipation.

▲ Ask your doctor, nurse, or nutritionist if you might need milk of magnesia or a magnesium supplement, a bowel regulator such as Metamucil or psyllium, or a laxative or stool softener.

▲ Get as much light exercise, such as walking, as your condition allows.

▲ Some pain medications can cause constipation. It's important to talk to your doctor, nurse, or nutritionist before this problem becomes serious.

DIARRHEA

▲ Call your doctor if you experience more than one episode of diarrhea a day, or if diarrhea is persistent.

▲ Stick to a clear-liquid diet for the next 12 to 14 hours after an acute bout of diarrhea.

▲ Drink liquids between meals, not during meals.

▲ Consume plenty of liquids and foods that contain sodium and potassium. These minerals are often lost when you have diarrhea. Bouillon or fat-free broth, bananas, peach or apricot nectar, and boiled or mashed potatoes are good choices.

▲ Limit beverages and foods that contain caffeine, such as coffee, strong tea, caffeinated sodas, and chocolate.

▲ Avoid greasy foods.

▲ Steer clear of foods with a high fiber content such as fresh fruits, fresh vegetables, and whole-grain cereals and breads.

▲ Consume foods warm or at room temperature.

▲ Drink tea and eat applesauce, baby foods, flavored gelatin, and toast. Cheese and cottage cheese are also good choices, but first rule out lactose intolerance as the cause of the diarrhea. Foods that are easy to digest and produce less residue will give the colon a chance to rest and heal.

▲ Eat small amounts throughout the day, rather than large meals.

SORE MOUTH OR THROAT

▲ Choose soft foods:
    Applesauce, bananas, watermelon, and other soft fruits
    Cottage cheese
    Custards, puddings, flavored gelatin
    Liquids
    Mashed potatoes, macaroni and cheese, or mashed sweet
        potatoes
    Milk shakes, or our Yogurt Protein Shake or Fresh Fruit

Smoothies. Tofu can be added to smoothies, or you can make tofu shakes.

Oatmeal or other cereals cooked in nonfat milk, or soy milk for added protein

Peach, pear, and apricot nectars

Puréed or mashed vegetables

Puréed meats, tofu, or beans

Scrambled eggs

▲ Purée food, using a blender or food processor.

▲ Cook foods until they are soft and tender, then cut into small pieces.

▲ Avoid rough, coarse, or dry foods such as raw vegetables and toast. Other foods that may irritate your mouth include citrus fruits or juices and spicy or salty foods.

▲ To make them easier to swallow, mix foods with low-fat yogurt, low-fat sour cream, or gravies and sauces made with fat-free broth and thickened with cornstarch.

▲ Eat foods cold or at room temperature rather than hot.

▲ Try tilting your head back or moving it forward while swallowing if you find that swallowing is difficult or painful.

▲ Drink plenty of fluids to avoid becoming dehydrated.

▲ Use a straw for drinking.

▲ Drink slippery elm tea if you find it soothing to your mouth and throat. It is available in tea bags at many grocery stores.

▲ For cleansing, mix a solution of 1 tablespoon of water and 1 tablespoon of hydrogen peroxide. Swish it around in your mouth and spit it out. **DO NOT SWALLOW IT.**

MANAGING TREATMENT RELATED SYMPTOMS

▲ Ask your doctor about anesthetic lozenges, sprays, or gargles that will numb your mouth and throat long enough for you to eat meals. Also, ask your doctor about using a mixture of equal parts viscous zylocaine, Maalox, and elixir of benedryl. This requires a prescription.

LACTOSE INTOLERANCE

Lactose intolerance means that your body can't digest milk sugar—*lactose*—found in milk products. Symptoms of this condition may include gas, diarrhea, and cramping after consuming dairy products. To minimize symptoms:

▲ Experiment with getting protein and calcium from sources other than milk products. Soybean formulas—such as soy milks and tofu, aged and reduced-fat cheeses and yogurt, or lactose-reduced or lactaid-type milks such as acidophilus milk—can often be consumed without symptoms occurring.

▲ Use fermented/cultured, reduced-fat milk products such as buttermilk, sour cream, and yogurt. They are often easier to digest than whole milk.

▲ Read labels carefully. Lactose is often a filler in products such as instant coffee and some medicines.

▲ Ask your doctor, nurse, or nutritionist about pills for lactose intolerance.

For many people, symptoms of lactose intolerance disappear a few weeks or months after treatment ends or when the intestine heals. Others will need to avoid dairy products indefinitely.

Loss of Appetite

▲ Don't panic. Your appetite will come back when you're feeling better.

▲ Eat whenever you are hungry. Several small meals throughout the day may work better for you than three big meals. Even a few bites of food or sips of liquid every hour or so can help you get the protein and calories you need.

▲ Plan your largest meals for breakfast or lunch if, like many cancer patients, your appetite is better earlier in the day. Try dinner foods at breakfast time and breakfast foods at dinnertime.

▲ Eat whatever sounds good. Remember that treatment is temporary and you can get back to making healthy choices when you feel better.

▲ Keep healthy, tasty snacks readily available.

▲ Drink plenty of fluids even if you can't eat much, so you don't become dehydrated.

▲ Add variety to your menu. Try new recipes and new ways of preparing old favorites.

▲ Arrange food attractively and create a pleasant environment. Eat with other people, if possible, or watch your favorite TV program while you eat.

▲ Eat off a small plate with small portions; a large plate with large portions can seem overwhelming. When you're eating out, ask for an extra plate, then spoon small portions onto it and eat from that. Or ask for half a portion.

▲ Don't hurry your meals. Relax and try to enjoy them.

▲ Talk to your doctor, nurse, or nutritionist about your symptoms.

LOSS OF WEIGHT

▲ Don't waste your appetite eating empty calories. You may want to ask for help from your nutritionist in choosing nutrient-rich foods you like.

▲ Select high-protein, nutrient-rich foods if you're being encouraged to eat lots of calories. For example, choose milk shakes made from soy milk and/or tofu instead of ice cream, peanut butter or almond butter instead of butter spread on bread or waffles, and avocado instead of mayonnaise in a sandwich or on toast.

▲ Add 2 teaspoons of dry skim milk powder per cup of milk called for in recipes to increase protein and calories without increasing fat content.

▲ Avoid drinking fluids before meals or filling up on soup or salad at the beginning of meals. Save your appetite for calorie-dense foods.

▲ Exercise about half an hour before meals to stimulate your appetite, but don't overdo it.

▲ Dine with friends or family members if possible. Most people eat more when they eat with other people than when they eat alone.

▲ Eat meals while you watch a favorite TV program or a great video. Distract your mind so you won't think about eating.

And, finally, a note to the caregiver: Keep a variety of foods available and offer them often. However, avoid urging food on the cancer patient. The person probably knows they have to eat and are doing the best they can. What's more, this may be the one area where they can exert some choice and control over their life.

WEIGHT GAIN

▲ Remember that with some cancers, such as breast cancer, it's common for people to gain weight with therapy. Be aware that there may be nothing you can do to control the weight gain. Dieting during treatment is generally not recommended.

▲ Consume plenty of water, six to eight glasses a day.

▲ Drink warm fluids such as tea or soup about 20 minutes before meals.

▲ Try six small meals a day rather than three big ones.

▲ Eat regularly instead of waiting until you are too hungry.

▲ Choose more high-fiber foods: fruits, vegetables, beans, and whole-grain cereals.

▲ Fill a small plate rather than a large one, to create the illusion that you're eating more than you are.

▲ Get as much exercise as your condition allows.

Fatigue

▲ Give yourself permission to let friends and family members help.

▲ Eat more when you're feeling well.

▲ Focus on eating high-protein, nutrient-rich foods.

▲ Avoid caffeine. It may give you a temporary lift, but there's a letdown. Gradually discontinue use of caffcine over a six-week period and you'll probably find you have more energy.

▲ Prepare and freeze meals ahead whenever possible. Label and date them before freezing.

▲ Give yourself permission to eat fast foods or prepared foods if that's all you can manage. While the goal is to eat healthy foods as often as possible, you may not always havc the energy to do that, and that's OK.

▲ Keep healthy snack foods—low-fat cheese and crackers, yogurt, fruit, vegetables, popcorn—readily accessible.

▲ Arrange for Meals on Wheels or a similar delivery service. Some grocery stores and restaurants will also make deliveries.

▲ Get extra rest.

▲ Experiment with breathing exercises, stress-reduction techniques, or meditation if you're having trouble relaxing or sleeping. Try watching funny movies. Call Cancer Lifeline or a similar organization for information about relaxation and stress-management classes in your area.

▲ Talk to your doctor if you're having trouble sleeping or relaxing; the problem may be treatable.

Changes in Sense of Taste

▲ Experiment with which foods taste best. Many people think that bland food is what they should be eating, but it's often the strong, spicy foods that sound and taste good. One person even reported craving sauerkraut.

▲ Marinate meat, fish, and chicken to intensify the flavor.

▲ Use more, or stronger, seasonings such as garlic, onion, and ginger to add flavor.

▲ Eat tart foods such as oranges or lemonade that may have more taste. Try our Lemon-Lime Fizz.

▲ Try new and different foods. While some of your favorite foods may not taste as good for a while, there's a good chance that *other* foods, even some you haven't liked in the past, will be appealing. Discover new favorites.

▲ Eat chicken, turkey, eggs, or dairy products—foods that don't have strong odors—rather than beef and pork.

▲ Use plastic utensils if you're bothered by a metallic taste.

GETTING THE HELP YOU NEED

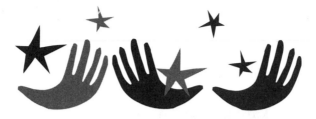

You may find that family and friends are eager to help, especially during the treatment process, but need some direction from you. On the other hand, maybe you're "going it alone" and need to find out about available resources. Here are a few suggestions.

PUTTING FRIENDS AND FAMILY TO WORK

The next time someone asks if there's anything they can do to help, ask them to do one or two of these tasks:

▲ Plan a week's worth of dinners.

▲ Accompany you to the grocery store.

▲ Take your list and go shopping for you.

▲ Help you prepare vegetables and other foods, or do it for you.

▲ Prepare a box of healthy, ready-to-eat snack foods.

▲ Organize friends and/or relatives to cook for you and your family. Each person might be responsible for making meals for one day. It works best if someone other than the cancer patient or caregiver organizes the effort. Meals should be delivered in either disposable containers or labeled so containers can be returned easily.

▲ Run errands, such as going to the cleaners, library, post office, or video store for you.

▲ Do a load of laundry or pay the bills.

▲ Vacuum your living room.

▲ Pick up the kids after school and take them on an enjoyable outing.

▲ Give the caregiver some time off.

▲ Take the patient or caregiver for a drive.

▲ Take the patient to a doctor's appointment.

▲ Listen.

GOING IT ALONE

▲ Call your church, the nurse at your doctor's office, a social worker, a community information line, or an organization like Cancer Lifeline to find out about services and resources that are available in your community. Services often include transportation, support groups, Meals on Wheels, a bookmobile, or help filling out insurance forms.

▲ Find a grocery store and some restaurants in your neighborhood that will deliver to your home.

▲ Organize your kitchen so foods are easy to find and within reach.

▲ Avoid buying food in hard-to-open containers or in cans if you can't use a can opener.

▲ Stock up on readily accessible snack foods such as almonds, walnuts, fresh fruit, bean dips, refried beans and tortillas, string cheese, and yogurt.

▲ Keep ready-to-eat prepared foods on hand for when you're feeling under the weather.

▲ Turn off the ringer on your phone when you want to rest, and turn on your answering machine.

▲ Make an effort not to become isolated.

▲ Reward yourself regularly. Order some flowers along with your groceries, treat yourself to a long-distance telephone call, or get a massage—whatever will give you some pleasure.

▲ Find new ways to incorporate rest, relaxation, and exercise into your life. Each activity may only last a few minutes, but it will help to invigorate you.

RECIPES FOR
HEALTHY EATING

APPLE PUFF

*This nutritious confection of whole grain and fruit
is light and sweet.*

SERVES 4

3 Granny Smith apples, peeled and sliced
1 teaspoon lemon juice
2 tablespoons "Better than Butter"
2 teaspoons cinnamon
1 tablespoon maple syrup
3 eggs
½ cup whole-wheat pastry flour
½ cup nonfat milk
1 teaspoon vanilla
dash of salt

1. Preheat oven to 450° F.
2. Sprinkle lemon juice over apples. In a frying pan, sauté apples
in "Better than Butter," cinnamon and syrup until soft.
3. Spread fruit over bottom of a 9" glass pie plate.
4. Beat eggs until frothy in a bowl. Add flour, beating until
smooth.
5. Stir in milk, vanilla and salt. Pour over apples.
6. Bake for 20 minutes or until lightly browned. Serve
immediately.

Per serving: Calories—219   Fat—8 gms   Protein—8 gms
Carbohydrates—32 gms   Fiber—4 gms   Sodium—145 mgs

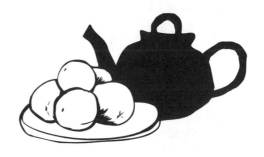

Blueberry Coffee Cake

*A high-fiber, low-fat version of an old breakfast
favorite, using whole-wheat and oat flours.*

SERVES 9

1 large egg
$\frac{1}{2}$ cup skim milk
$\frac{1}{2}$ cup plain nonfat yogurt
3 tablespoons "Better than Butter"
$\frac{1}{2}$ cup oat flour
1 cup whole-wheat pastry flour
$\frac{1}{2}$ cup all-purpose unbleached flour
$\frac{1}{2}$ cup sugar
4 teaspoons baking powder
$\frac{1}{2}$ teaspoon salt
$1\frac{1}{2}$ cups fresh or frozen unsweetened blueberries
3 tablespoons sugar
2 tablespoons finely chopped walnuts
$\frac{1}{4}$ teaspoon cinnamon

1. Preheat oven to 400° F.
2. Coat an 8" square baking pan with nonstick cooking spray.
3. In a large mixing bowl, whisk together egg, milk, yogurt and "Better than Butter."
4. Mix flours, $\frac{1}{2}$ cup sugar, baking powder and salt in a bowl.
5. Sift dry ingredients into liquid mixture.
6. Stir batter just to blend. Do not overbeat.
7. Fold in blueberries and turn batter into prepared pan.
8. In a small bowl, stir together 3 tablespoons sugar, walnuts and cinnamon. Sprinkle over batter.
9. Bake cake for 20 to 25 minutes or until top is golden brown and a knife inserted into center of cake comes out clean.
10. Cool on a rack for 10 minutes. Cut into squares and serve warm.

Per serving: Calories—214   Fat—4 gms   Protein—6 gms
Carbohydrates—40 gms   Fiber—3 gms   Sodium—374 mgs

BREAKFAST BURRITO

Breakfast burritos - scrambled eggs and beans wrapped in a tortilla and topped with salsa, sour cream or plain yogurt - are simple to make and delicious. They are quickly becoming a popular breakfast item.

SERVES 4

2 teaspoons olive oil
$\frac{1}{2}$ cup onion, chopped
$\frac{1}{2}$ green or red bell pepper, chopped
2 cloves garlic, minced
$\frac{1}{2}$ teaspoon cumin
1 15-ounce can nonfat refried beans
4 eggs, beaten
4 whole-wheat tortillas
$\frac{1}{4}$ cup low-fat sour cream
$\frac{1}{4}$ cup nonfat plain yogurt
salsa

1. Preheat oven to 350° F.
2. In a large skillet, heat olive oil over medium heat.
3. Add onions, bell pepper and garlic. Sauté until tender. Add cumin.
4. Warm beans in a saucepan.
5. Whisk eggs, then pour over sautéed vegetables. Carefully stir until eggs are soft and well scrambled.
6. Heat tortillas in oven for about 10 minutes.
7. Fill each tortilla with a quarter of the eggs and beans. Top with choice of yogurt or sour cream. Add salsa to taste.

Per serving: Calories—361   Fat—10 gms   Protein—20 gms
Carbohydrates—54 gms   Fiber—12 gms   Sodium—623 mgs

CLAFOUTI
FRUIT AND EGG BAKE

Kids love this weekend breakfast treat that is fairly low in fat and high in protein. Fruit never tasted quite so good before.

SERVES 4 TO 6

1½ cups nonfat milk
3 eggs
3 egg whites
¾ cup whole-wheat pastry flour
¾ cup all-purpose unbleached flour
1 teaspoon vanilla
3 tablespoons brown sugar
¼ teaspoon salt
2 cups fruit - fresh, frozen or canned (drained) cherries, blue-berries, blackberries, peaches or any combination

1. Preheat oven to 375° F.
2. Combine all ingredients except fruit in a blender. Blend for at least 2 minutes until frothy.
3. Coat a 9 x 13" pan with cooking spray and pour in egg batter.
4. Evenly spoon fruit over batter.
5. Bake for 35 minutes or until puffy and lightly browned.
6. Serve with powdered sugar.

Per serving: Calories—266 Fat—4 gms Protein—13 gms
Carbohydrates—46 gms Fiber—4 gms Sodium—223 mgs

FRESH FRUIT SMOOTHIES

David deVarona, owner of Todo Loco Restaurants, Seattle

These combinations of fresh fruit, nonfat yogurt and ice are blended into cool, smooth and nutritious drinks. They are great for breakfast, dessert or snacks. You can turn any of these into an Energy Boost Smoothie by adding 1 teaspoon of spirulina, protein powder, or bee pollen. Once you've mastered the basics, have some fun trying your own variations with your favorite fruits.

SERVES 1

PEACHES AND CREAM

$\frac{1}{2}$ cup ice
1 peach, peeled, pitted and quartered
1 banana
2 tablespoons nonfat frozen vanilla yogurt
orange juice

1. Place ice, fruits and frozen yogurt in blender. Add juice to the 16-ounce line on blender container.
2. Blend all ingredients until smooth.

PINEAPPLE PLEASURE

$\frac{1}{2}$ cup ice
2 spears pineapple, about $\frac{1}{4}$ of fresh, peeled pineapple
1 banana
$\frac{1}{4}$ cup nonfat frozen vanilla yogurt
orange juice

1. Place ice, fruits and frozen yogurt in blender. Add juice to the 16-ounce line on blender container.
2. Blend all ingredients until smooth.

VERY STRAWBERRY

½ cup ice
½ cup fresh or frozen strawberries
1 banana
¼ cup nonfat frozen vanilla yogurt
apple juice

1. Place ice, fruits and frozen yogurt in blender. Add juice to the 16-ounce line on blender container.
2. Blend all ingredients until smooth.

Per serving: Calories—217 Fat—1 gm Protein—4 gms
Carbohydrates—53 gms Fiber—4 gms Sodium—23 mgs

MUESLI

Muesli is a great comfort food that is easily digested and provides sustained energy. Fresh peaches, nectarines or berries may be served alongside.

SERVES 4

1½ cups old-fashioned rolled oats
1½ cups nonfat milk
1½ tablespoons lemon juice
2 grated Granny Smith or Fuji apples
¼ cup nuts, finely chopped, such as almonds or walnuts
1 tablespoon raisins
½ teaspoon cinnamon

1. Combine oats and milk in a large bowl. Let stand 15 minutes.
2. Sprinkle lemon juice over apples, then drain.
3. Stir fruit into oat mixture.
4. Spoon into individual serving bowls and sprinkle with an assortment of nuts and/or raisins. Add a dash of cinnamon.

Per serving: Calories—239 Fat—7 gms Protein—10 gms
Carbohydrates—38 gms Fiber—5 gms Sodium—50 mgs

VERY FRENCH TOAST

A rich and delicious variation on an old favorite, this "very French toast" is even better if the batter is prepared ahead and refrigerated overnight.

SERVES 4

$1/4$ cup nonfat milk
$1/3$ cup freshly squeezed orange juice
1 tablespoon Grand Marnier, optional, or 1 teaspoon grated
  orange peel or $1/2$ teaspoon orange extract
1 tablespoon brown sugar
$1/4$ teaspoon cinnamon
$1/4$ teaspoon vanilla
4 eggs
8 slices whole-grain bread, sliced thick
4 teaspoons powdered sugar

1. Combine milk, orange juice, Grand Marnier, sugar, cinnamon, vanilla and eggs. Beat until smooth. If desired, refrigerate overnight.
2. Soak bread in egg mixture.
3. Coat a nonstick frying pan with cooking spray and add bread. Cook on medium heat about 3 to 4 minutes a side or until golden brown. Continue coating pan as needed when adding bread.
4. Sprinkle with powdered sugar before serving.

Per serving: Calories—283   Fat—7.5 gms   Protein—12.5 gms
Carbohydrates—42 gms   Fiber—4.5 gms   Sodium—441 mgs

WHOLE-GRAIN PANCAKES OR WAFFLES

Full of fiber and not much fat, these versatile pancakes are sure to enjoy wide appeal. Other whole grains such as oat bran, oat flour, amaranth flour, cornmeal, rolled oats or buckwheat flour may be substituted for whole-wheat flour. Consider adding fruit, nuts or sunflower seeds.

SERVES 6

2 cups whole-wheat pastry flour
3 teaspoons baking powder
$1/2$ teaspoon salt
1 tablespoon sweetener (brown or date sugar or fruit concentrate)
3 eggs, separated, or 2 whites and 2 whole eggs
2 cups nonfat buttermilk or soy milk (for waffles, reduce to $1\frac{1}{4}$ cups)
1 tablespoon "Better than Butter"

1. Preheat a lightly greased frying pan.
2. Sift together all dry ingredients in a large mixing bowl. Set aside.
3. Beat egg yolks, buttermilk and "Better than Butter." Mix in dry ingredients until just moist.
4. Beat egg whites into stiff peaks and gently fold into batter.
5. Using a $1/4$ cup measure, drop batter onto frying pan, spacing pancakes well apart. Cook until golden brown on each side.

Per serving: Calories—225   Fat—5 gms   Protein—11 gms
Carbohydrates—36 gms   Fiber—5 gms   Sodium—548 mgs

YOGURT PROTEIN SHAKE

A refreshing, high-protein shake that is loaded with vitamins, minerals and fiber and is great for breakfast - or any time. Frozen fruit gives the shake a consistency similar to that of an ice cream shake. For variety, substitute vanilla-flavored soy milk for any milk or fruit juice called for in the following recipes; add 2 ounces soft, silken-style tofu for extra protein, carbohydrates and fiber.

SERVES 1

$^1/_2$ cup nonfat yogurt
$1^1/_2$ teaspoons protein powder (any made with whey, soy or egg is acceptable)
$^1/_2$ cup fresh or frozen fruit, such as cherries, peaches, melon or berries
1 banana, fresh or frozen
$^1/_4$ cup or more fruit juice, depending upon desired consistency
1 to 2 dates, pitted (optional)

Combine in a blender, mixing until smooth.

Per serving: Calories—294   Fat—2 gms   Protein—10 gms
Carbohydrates—65 gms Fiber—5 gm   Sodium—110 mgs

VARIATIONS
CHERRY SHAKE

$^1/_2$–$^3/_4$ cup sweet frozen cherries, pitted
$^1/_3$ cup Knudsen's cherry juice
$1^1/_2$ teaspoons protein powder
1 banana, sliced
$^1/_2$ cup nonfat yogurt
2 dates, pitted (optional)

Strawberry Shake

$\frac{1}{2}$ cup strawberry nonfat yogurt
$\frac{1}{2}$ cup frozen strawberries
$\frac{1}{2}$ cup apple juice
1 banana, sliced
$1\frac{1}{2}$ teaspoons protein powder
2 dates, pitted

Extra Calorie Shake

Add $\frac{1}{2}$ to 1 tablespoon flaxseed oil to any of the shakes. This also increases the fat grams by 6 to 11 grams, respectively.

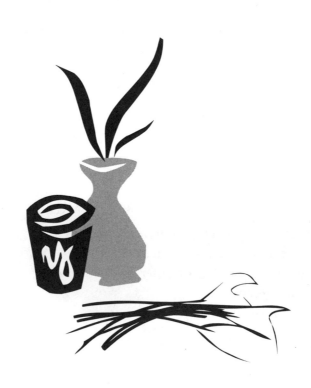

Potato Rolls

This versatile recipe is also the basis for our Cinnamon Rolls (see page 88).

Makes 18 to 20 rolls

1 large potato, peeled and cut into quarters
$\frac{1}{2}$ cup "Better than Butter"
$\frac{1}{4}$ cup sugar
2 teaspoons salt
1 package active dry yeast (or 2 teaspoons)
2 eggs
$3\frac{1}{2}$ to 4 cups all-purpose unbleached flour
$3\frac{1}{2}$ to 4 cups whole-wheat pastry flour

1. In a saucepan, cook potato until soft in enough boiling water to cover. Drain, reserving $1\frac{1}{2}$ cups hot cooking liquid. Add "Better than Butter," sugar and salt to liquid and stir until dissolved.
2. Allow liquid to cool until lukewarm (about 115° F.), then stir in yeast until dissolved. Let stand 5 minutes. Meanwhile, mash the potato.
3. Using a wooden spoon, stir in eggs, 1 cup mashed potato and 2 cups unbleached flour. Stir in 2 cups whole-wheat flour. Gradually stir in remaining flour.
4. Place on a floured surface and knead by hand until dough is no longer sticky, approximately 10 minutes. Cover with a damp towel and let rise in a warm place until double in size.
5. Punch down dough. Break off small handfuls of dough and roll each in your hands to size of medium lemon — about 2" in diameter. You should have 18 to 20 when done. Place on lightly greased baking sheet about 1" apart.
6. Let rise again until double in size.
7. Bake at 400° F. for 20 minutes or until golden brown.

Per roll: Calories—264   Fat—5 gms   Protein—8 gms
Carbohydrates—48 gms   Fiber—4 gms   Sodium—313 mgs

BUTTERMILK BISCUITS

These biscuits are easy to make and take only a short time to prepare. They require no rising. For a nice brown crust, brush the tops with milk or butter.

MAKES 10 TO 12 BISCUITS

1⅓ cups all-purpose unbleached flour
⅔ cup whole-wheat pastry flour
1 tablespoon cornmeal
1 tablespoon baking powder
1 teaspoon baking soda
½ teaspoon salt
1 cup fresh buttermilk (reconstituted dry buttermilk may be substituted)
⅓ cup "Better than Butter"

1. Preheat oven to 375° F.
2. Mix together flour, cornmeal, baking powder, baking soda and salt.
3. Add buttermilk and "Better than Butter." Mix until moist.
4. Turn dough onto lightly floured board.
5. Knead gently for about a minute.
6. Roll dough into an oval, 1" thick.
7. Using biscuit cutter (or rim of glass dipped in flour), cut into biscuits and place on a cookie sheet.
8. Bake for 15 minutes or until golden brown.

Per biscuit: Calories—132 Fat—4 gms Protein—4 gms
Carbohydrates—21 gms Fiber—2 gms Sodium—424 mgs

Hint: Mix an extra batch of dry ingredients together and store in airtight container. The following is enough for three batches.

4 cups all-purpose unbleached flour
2 cups whole-wheat pastry flour
3 tablespoons cornmeal
3 tablespoons baking powder
3 teaspoons baking soda
1$\frac{1}{2}$ teaspoons salt

When you're ready to make more biscuits, moisten 2 cups plus 2 tablespoons of the dry mix with 1 cup buttermilk and $\frac{1}{3}$ cup "Better than Butter" and proceed with the rest of the directions.

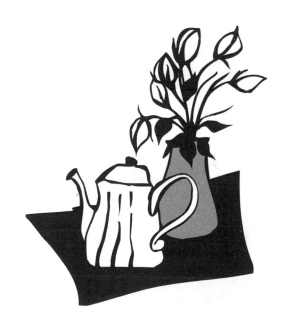

OAT AND DATE SCONES

Scones are traditionally richer than regular biscuits due to the butter and egg. However, these scones are filled with whole grains and fiber, and also include oat flour. A teaspoon of finely grated orange peel or a half cup of dried apricots may be substituted for the dates.

MAKES 8

1 cup all-purpose unbleached flour
$\frac{1}{2}$ cup whole-wheat pastry flour
$\frac{1}{2}$ cup oat flour (Place oatmeal in the blender and grind for a
  minute or so)
4 tablespoons brown sugar
2 teaspoons baking powder
$\frac{1}{2}$ teaspoon baking soda
$\frac{1}{2}$ cup "Better than Butter"
$\frac{1}{2}$ cup chopped dates
1 egg, lightly whisked
$\frac{1}{2}$ cup buttermilk

1. Preheat oven to 375° F.
2. In a large mixing bowl, combine flour, sugar, baking powder and baking soda.
3. Using a fork, blend in "Better than Butter" until mixture is crumbly. Stir in dates.
4. Add egg and buttermilk, stirring with a fork until dough holds together.
5. Gently knead dough a few times on a lightly floured board. Do not overmix. Add up to 2 tablespoons more flour if dough seems too sticky to work with.
6. Shape dough into an 8" round. Cut into 8 wedges and arrange on a nonstick baking sheet 2" apart.
7. Bake for 20 minutes or until golden brown. Serve warm.

Per serving: Calories—234   Fat—8 gms   Protein—5 gms
Carbohydrates—37 gms   Fiber—3 gms   Sodium—262 mgs

CORN BREAD

A wholesome bread that stands out on its own or complements soups and salads. It is especially good warm. Stone-ground cornmeal will give the bread a crunchier texture.

SERVES 8

Hint: For a crispy crust, preheat pan or muffin tins in the heated oven before filling.

$\frac{1}{2}$ cup all-purpose unbleached white flour
1 cup cornmeal
$\frac{1}{2}$ cup whole-wheat pastry flour
2 tablespoons brown sugar
1 tablespoon baking powder
$\frac{3}{4}$ cup nonfat milk
$\frac{1}{2}$ cup onion, finely chopped (optional)
1 8-ounce can cream-style corn
2 tablespoons "Better than Butter"
1 teaspoon low-sodium soy sauce
1 egg

1. Preheat oven to 400° F.
2. Sift all dry ingredients into a large bowl.
3. In a separate bowl, blend milk, onion, corn, "Better then Butter," soy sauce and egg.
4. Pour milk mixture into flour mixture, stirring briskly until just moist.
5. Pour batter into greased 9 x 9" pan or large muffin tin.
6. Bake for 25 to 30 minutes.

Per serving: Calories—187 Fat—3 gms Protein—6 gms
Carbohydrates—36 gms Fiber—3 gms Sodium—320 mgs

CINNAMON ROLLS

A sweet breakfast treat you'll enjoy any time.

MAKES 12 ROLLS

1 recipe Potato Rolls dough (see page 83)
3 tablespoons "Better than Butter," melted
½ cup date sugar
½ cup brown sugar
1 tablespoon cinnamon
½ cup nuts and/or ⅓ cup raisins (optional)

1. Preheat oven to 400° F.
2. Prepare Potato Rolls through step 5.
3. Punch down dough and roll out to ¼" thick rectangle 24" long.
4. Brush dough with "Better than Butter".
5. Mix together date sugar, brown sugar and cinnamon and sprinkle on dough. Add nuts and raisins if desired.
6. Roll up into a log about 2 feet long. Cut into 2" slices.
7. Place slices 2" apart on buttered baking sheet. Let rise until doubled and bake 20 minutes or until golden brown.

Per roll: Calories—410   Fat—8 gms   Protein—10 gms
Carbohydrates—78 gms   Fiber—7 gms   Sodium—404 mgs

BLACK-EYED PEAS AND HAM SOUP

Any type of bean may be used in making this easy one-pot meal, but black-eyed peas lend a distinctive flavor. For a complete meal, serve the soup with a side of corn bread. Hint: To reduce cooking time, canned beans may be substituted.

SERVES 4

1 cup dry black-eyed peas or one 15-ounce can of canned beans
4 cups water
2 cups low-sodium chicken broth
4 cups water
$3/4$ pound nitrate-free ham hocks (optional)
1 onion, chopped
2 stalks celery, chopped
2 cloves garlic, minced
$1/2$ teaspoon pepper
1 bunch fresh kale, collard greens or other green leafy
   vegetable, chopped
1 strip dried Kombu seaweed (optional)

1. Bring 4 cups water to a boil and add peas. Return water to a boil, then remove peas from heat and drain. When using canned beans, omit step 1 and reduce the amount of water to 2 cups in step 2.
2. Combine peas with all remaining ingredients except greens and bring to a boil. Reduce heat and simmer for $1\frac{1}{2}$ hours. Add greens and cook for another $1/2$ hour or until tender.

Note: If adding ham hocks, be sure to remove bone and skin after cooking. For less fat, refrigerate finished soup overnight and remove congealed fat. Heat well before serving.

Per serving: Calories—389   Fat—14 gms   Protein—30 gms
Carbohydrates—36 gms   Fiber—7 gms   Sodium—287 mgs

CARROT SOUP

Chef Jacques, of Queen Anne Thriftway and KIRO-TV, Seattle

A soup that is naturally good.

SERVES 4

4 tablespoons "Better than Butter"
1 small onion, chopped
2 cloves garlic, crushed
1 pound fresh carrots, cut into pieces
8 cups low sodium chicken broth or chicken stock
salt and pepper to taste
nonfat yogurt or "Better than Butter"

1. Heat "Better than Butter" in a large stockpot until it starts to foam. Add onion and garlic and cook until clear.
2. Add carrots and chicken stock. Simmer until carrots are soft.
3. Purée soup in a processor until smooth. Add salt and pepper to taste. Serve topped with a dollop of yogurt or 1 teaspoon "Better than Butter."

Per serving: Calories—193   Fat—9 gms   Protein—12 gms
Carbohydrates—15 gms   Fiber—3 gms   Sodium—160 mgs

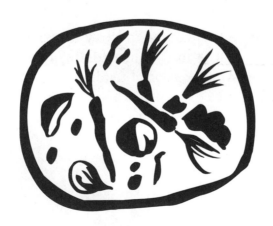

CHICKEN SOUP WITH CAULIFLOWER & GREEN BEANS

Packed with vegetables, this basic soup is sure to please.

SERVES 4 TO 6

1 quart water
1 15-ounce can low sodium chicken broth
flowerettes of 1 cauliflower
1 10-ounce package frozen green beans
1 to 2 cups cooked rice or cooked fine noodles
2 chicken bouillon cubes (optional)

1. Heat water and chicken broth to a boil. Add vegetables and
cook until tender.
2. Add rice or noodles and simmer for 15 minutes.
3. Add bouillon cubes for extra flavor. Season to taste.

Per serving: Calories—123 Fat—1 gm Protein—5 gms
Carbohydrates—23 gms Fiber—3 gms Sodium—496 mgs

CHILLED AVOCADO SOUP

Chef Jacques, of Queen Anne Thriftway and KIRO-TV, Seattle

This soup with salsa doubles as a wonderful sauce for any grilled fish such as salmon, halibut or ling cod. Remember, avocados are a good source of monounsaturated fat.

SERVES 4

Tomato Salsa (recipe follows)
2 avocados, peeled and pit removed
1 clove garlic
2 cups chicken stock, chilled
1 cup clam juice, chilled
1 stalk celery, chopped

1. Prepare Tomato Salsa.
2. Using a food processor, blend remaining ingredients until smooth.
3. Ladle into bowls and top with dollop of Tomato Salsa.

TOMATO SALSA

1 cup tomatoes, diced
1 teaspoon red onion, minced
1 teaspoon cilantro, minced
2 tablespoons vinegar
salt and chilies to taste

Combine all ingredients in a small bowl. Makes about 1 cup.

Per serving: Calories—199 Fat—16 gms   Protein—5 gms
Carbohydrates—12 gms   Fiber—5 gms Sodium—540 mgs

COUNTRY LENTIL SOUP

Chef Jacques, of Queen Anne Thriftway and KIRO-TV, Seattle

*This tasty soup can be prepared ahead, and is
even better when reheated.*

SERVES 6

2 cups dry lentils
2 tablespoons olive oil
1 medium onion, chopped
4 cloves garlic, minced
1 celery stalk, diced
1 carrot, diced
8 cups water
1 sprig thyme
1 bay leaf
2 sprigs parsley
$\frac{1}{2}$ teaspoon ground cumin
salt and pepper to taste
4 tablespoons wine vinegar
pita bread

1. Soak lentils in cold water overnight. Drain well and discard soaking water.
2. Heat olive oil in a large stockpot. Add onion, garlic, celery and carrot. Sauté until golden brown.
3. Add drained lentils and 8 cups water to the pot. Add thyme, bay leaf, parsley, cumin, salt and pepper. Bring to a boil. Reduce heat, and simmer for 1 to 1½ hours.
4. Stir in vinegar. Serve accompanied with warm pita bread.

Per serving: Calories—275   Fat—5 gms   Protein—19 gms
Carbohydrates—41 gms   Fiber—9 gms   Sodium—28 mgs

"CREAM" OF BROCCOLI SOUP

A low-fat soup that's bursting with flavor. It's easy to make and any leftovers keep well in the refrigerator.

SERVES 6 TO 8

2 stems broccoli
4 cups chicken broth
2 tablespoons "Better than Butter"
$\frac{1}{2}$ medium onion, chopped
2 tablespoons whole-wheat pastry flour
2 cups nonfat milk
4 ounces part-skim mozzarella
1 teaspoon salt (may be omitted if chicken broth is salted)
$\frac{1}{2}$ teaspoon curry powder

1. Cook broccoli in chicken broth about 20 minutes until tender.
2. Melt "Better than Butter" in a medium skillet. Sauté onion for about 5 minutes until transparent.
3. Add flour. Stir until blended, then pour in milk. Continue stirring until well heated and mixture thickens slightly.
4. Remove from heat and thoroughly blend in cheese, curry powder and salt.
5. Add stock to cheese sauce. Pour in small batches into the food processor and blend slightly. Leave broccoli coarsely chopped.
6. May be reheated to serve, but be careful not to boil.

Per serving: Calories—131   Fat—6 gms   Protein—11 gms
Carbohydrates—9 gms   Fiber—2 gms   Sodium—586 mgs

"CREAM" OF RED PEPPER SOUP

A satisfying, sweet soup that is low in fat. Its smooth texture and creamy taste are especially appealing.

SERVES 4 TO 6

1 tablespoon "Better than Butter"
2 cups minced onion
1 tablespoon garlic, crushed
1 teaspoon salt
pinch of freshly ground black pepper
$\frac{1}{2}$ teaspoon cumin
5 medium red bell peppers, thinly sliced
1 tablespoon whole-wheat pastry flour
$\frac{1}{2}$ cup chicken stock or water
$2\frac{1}{2}$ cups nonfat milk
nonfat yogurt
cilantro
basil

1. Melt "Better than Butter" in a large pot.
2. Gently sauté onions and garlic with salt, pepper and cumin for about 5 minutes or until soft and clear.
3. Stir in bell peppers.
4. Cover and cook over low heat for 10 to 15 minutes, stirring frequently.
5. Gradually sprinkle in flour. Cook for 5 minutes longer.
6. Add stock or water, cover and cook another 2 to 3 minutes. Remove from heat.
7. Purée soup in small amounts while gradually adding milk. Return soup to the pot and heat very gently. Do not boil. Serve topped with yogurt. Sprinkle with fresh cilantro or basil to taste.

Per serving: Calories—107   Fat—2 gms   Protein—6 gms
Carbohydrates—18 gms   Fiber—3 gms   Sodium—501 mgs

HEARTY LENTIL TOMATO SOUP

A robust cold weather soup brimming with vegetables.
Serve it with fresh bread and green salad.

SERVES 8

1 cup carrots, thinly sliced
1 cup onion, chopped
1 cup celery, chopped
2 cloves garlic, chopped
1 tablespoon olive oil
2 cups water
2 14-ounce cans low-sodium chicken broth
1 8-ounce can low-sodium tomato sauce
1 cup dried lentils, uncooked
½ teaspoon ground cumin seed
½ teaspoon coarsely ground pepper

1. Using a large pot, sauté carrots, onion, celery and garlic in olive oil over medium heat.
2. Add water, chicken broth and tomato sauce. Stir well.
3. Add lentils and seasonings. Bring to a boil. Reduce heat, cover and let simmer for about 1½ hours or more, until lentils are tender. For a smoother texture, purée the soup before serving.

Per serving: Calories—138 Fat—3 gms Protein—10 gms
Carbohydrates—20 gms Fiber—5 gms Sodium—59 mgs

Josephine's Chicken Soup

Chef Jacques, of Queen Anne Thriftway and KIRO-TV, Seattle

Always comforting for whatever the ailment!

Serves 6

2 to 3 pound stewing chicken
2 sprigs fresh parsley
1 bay leaf
4 small carrots, pared and cut into pieces
4 stalks celery, cut into pieces
1 small onion, cut into pieces
1 parsnip, pared and cut into pieces
6 matzoh balls (follow directions on matzoh meal package)
salt and freshly ground pepper to taste

1. Place chicken, parsley, bay leaf and vegetables in a large Dutch oven. Add water to cover, bring to a boil and simmer 1½ hours or until chicken is tender.
2. Remove chicken with a slotted spoon. Remove skin and meat from bones. Cut meat into bite-size pieces.
3. Return chicken meat to pot. Allow stock to cool slightly before refrigerating overnight. Remove any solidified fat.
4. Make matzoh balls, forming balls approximately 1" in diameter.
5. Reheat stock to a boil, add matzoh balls and seasonings. Simmer until heated through. Serve very hot in deep soup plates with unleavened crackers.

Per serving: Calories—256   Fat—13 gms   Protein—25 gms
Carbohydrates—10 gms   Fiber—2 gms   Sodium—101 mgs

Mom's Mushroom Soup

*This sweet and creamy soup is an old Czechoslovakian treasure.
The fat content has been reduced from the traditional recipe
by using nonfat and low-fat dairy products.*

Serves 5 to 6

1 cup onion, chopped
½ cup red pepper, chopped
4 cloves garlic, minced
4 tablespoons "Better than Butter"
1 cup fresh mushrooms, sliced
1 cup fresh shiitake mushrooms, washed and sliced
1 tablespoon low-sodium soy sauce
1 tablespoon dill weed
1 tablespoon sweet Hungarian paprika
2 cups low-sodium chicken broth
4 tablespoons whole-wheat pastry flour
1 cup nonfat milk
1 cup low-fat sour cream
2 teaspoons lemon juice

1. In a saucepan, sauté onions, red pepper and garlic in 2 tablespoons of "Better than Butter" until tender.
2. Add mushrooms, soy sauce, dill, paprika and 1 cup broth. Cover and simmer for 20 minutes.
3. Melt 2 tablespoons of "Better than Butter" in a large soup pot. Whisk in flour and cook for 3 minutes, stirring constantly. Slowly add milk and the remaining cup of broth. Continue to stir over medium heat for another 10 minutes.
4. Stir in the mushroom mixture. Cover and cook gently for 15 minutes.
5. Blend in sour cream and lemon juice and serve.

Per serving: Calories—171 Fat—2 gms Protein—6 gms
Carbohydrates—16 gms Fiber—2 gms Sodium—188 mgs

QUICK BLACK BEAN SOUP

This tasty soup is packed with five of the Top 10 "Super Foods" - cruciferous vegetables, beans, shiitake mushrooms, yogurt and garlic - and only takes about half an hour to prepare.

SERVES 6

$\frac{1}{2}$ onion, chopped
2 cloves garlic, chopped
2 stalks celery, chopped
2 leaves kale or bok choy, finely chopped
2 fresh shiitake mushrooms, cut into small pieces
$\frac{1}{2}$ teaspoon cumin, or to taste
2 15-ounce cans low-sodium chicken broth
2 15-ounce cans low-sodium black beans
3 cups water
low-fat plain yogurt
parsley, chopped

1. Cook onion, garlic, celery, kale or bok choy, mushrooms and cumin in 2 tablespoons of chicken broth in a large nonstick skillet for about 10 minutes or until soft.
2. Add remaining broth, beans and water. Simmer for 20 minutes.
3. Pour soup into bowls and top with yogurt and parsley.

Per serving: Calories—226   Fat—2 gms   Protein—16 gms
Carbohydrates—38 gms   Fiber—13 gms   Sodium—64 mgs

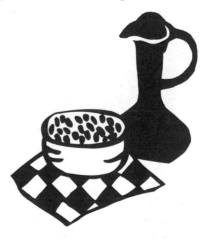

SQUASH SOUP

A soup that is sure to ward off the autumn chill.

SERVES 4

1 onion, diced
1 tablespoon olive oil
½ cup oatmeal
2 teaspoons dried basil
5 cups chicken stock
¼ teaspoon ground cloves
2 pounds butternut or acorn squash, peeled and diced
2 tablespoons cilantro, minced

1. In a medium-size saucepan, sauté onion in olive oil until transparent.
2. Add oatmeal and basil and "roast" for 2 to 3 minutes, stirring constantly. Pour in chicken stock.
3. Add cloves and squash and bring to a boil. Reduce heat and simmer for 15 to 20 minutes or until squash is tender.
4. Purée in a blender.
5. Stir in cilantro before serving.

Per serving: Calories—123   Fat—1 gm   Protein—5 gms
Carbohydrates—23 gms   Fiber—3 gms   Sodium—496 mgs

TOFU MISO SOUP

A simple soup that combines the nutritious properties of tofu with the rich flavor of miso. Miso is a paste made from grains and fermented soybeans. It comes in red, brown or yellow varieties, depending upon the type of grain that has been added to the soybeans. This recipe calls for brown miso, which is made with barley.

SERVES 4

3" strip dried Kombu or Wakame seaweed
3½ cups water
½ cup grated carrot
½ cup bok choy or kale, chopped
¼ cup green onion, finely sliced
½ cup reduced fat, silken firm tofu, cubed
1 tablespoon brown miso

1. Allow dried seaweed to soak in ½ cup of water for 5 minutes. Cut seaweed into small pieces with scissors.
2. Bring 3 cups of water to a boil in a large pot.
3. Add seaweed and carrots and simmer for 5 minutes.
4. Stir in bok choy or kale and cook on medium heat for 5 minutes.
5. Add green onion and tofu and simmer for 5 minutes.
6. Turn off heat. Gently dissolve miso into soup, taking care not to boil.

Per serving: Calories—43   Fat—2 gms   Protein—3 gms
Carbohydrates—4 gms   Fiber—1 gm   Sodium—186 mgs

VEGETABLE SOUP WITH LEEKS

Chef Jacques, of Queen Anne Thriftway and KIRO-TV, Seattle

This soup is served in many French homes during the winter months. The vegetables can vary with availability. The leek, a member of the lily family (and related to onion), is also called the "poor man's asparagus." Serve with a crusty loaf of French bread.

SERVES 4

2 large carrots
2 leeks
2 medium potatoes
2 medium turnips
1 sprig fresh thyme
10 cups cold water, or 5 cups low-sodium chicken broth and
   5 cups cold water
"Better than Butter" (optional)
salt and pepper
French bread

1. Peel and wash all vegetables. Cut into small pieces.
2. Place vegetables in a large cooking pot with thyme. Add water, bring to a boil and simmer 30 to 45 minutes or until vegetables are soft.
3. Purée the soup in a food processor or food mill. Add salt and pepper to taste. Serve in warm soup plates topped with a tablespoon of "Better then Butter."

Per serving: Calories—131 Fat—0 gms Protein—3 gms
Carbohydrates—30 gms Fiber—5 gms Sodium—96 mgs

BLACK & WHITE BEAN SALAD

A colorful, crunchy salad with a zesty appeal.

SERVES 4

1 15-ounce can low-sodium cannellini, navy or white beans, drained and rinsed
1 15-ounce can low-sodium black beans, drained and rinsed
1¼ cups peeled, seeded and chopped tomatoes
¾ cup diced red bell pepper
¾ cup diced yellow bell pepper
¾ cup green onions, thinly sliced
½ cup low-sodium salsa
¼ cup red wine vinegar
2 tablespoons chopped fresh cilantro
⅛ teaspoon freshly ground black pepper
¼ to ½ teaspoon ground cumin seed to taste

1. In a large bowl, gently mix beans and chopped tomato.
2. Add peppers and green onions. Set aside.
3. Combine salsa, vinegar, cilantro, pepper and cumin in a small bowl and stir with a wire whisk until well blended. Pour over beans and toss lightly.
4. Line a large serving bowl with shredded lettuce and fill with salad.

Per serving: Calories—274   Fat—1 gm   Protein—18 gms
Carbohydrates—51 gms   Fiber—15 gms   Sodium—137 mgs

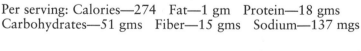
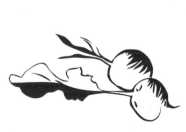
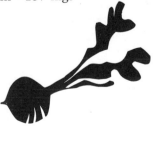

GARDEN VEGETABLE MEDLEY

Chef Jacques, of Queen Anne Thriftway and KIRO-TV, Seattle

A delightful combination of fresh vegetables.

SERVES 6

3 tablespoons olive oil
2 cloves garlic, minced
16 pearl onions, peeled
1 cup water
24 baby carrots, peeled
2 sprigs thyme
24 green string beans, trimmed
2 cups fresh green peas, shelled
1 head Bibb lettuce, leaves separated and cleaned
1 tablespoon chervil or parsley, chopped
2 tablespoons nonfat yogurt
salt and pepper

1. Heat olive oil in a large saucepan over medium heat. Sauté garlic and onions. Add water, carrots, thyme and a pinch of salt. Cover tightly and simmer for 15 minutes.
2. Stir in green beans and peas. Cover and simmer for 10 minutes or until tender. Make sure there is enough liquid in the pan. Add water if necessary.
3. Just prior to serving, add lettuce leaves. Toss quickly over high heat until wilted. Top with herbs and yogurt. Add salt and pepper.

Per serving: Calories—164   Fat—7 gms   Protein—5 gms
Carbohydrates—22 gms   Fiber—8 gms   Sodium—120 mgs

Green Beans and Mushroom Salad

Chef Jacques, of Queen Anne Thriftway and KIRO-TV, Seattle

This slightly tart vinaigrette enhances the flavor of fresh vegetables. Serve with a crusty loaf of French bread.

SERVES 4

1 pound fresh green beans
6 white mushrooms, thinly sliced
1 fresh tomato, sliced
Piquant Dijon Vinaigrette (recipe follows)

1. Snap off green bean ends. Blanch beans in boiling, salted water for 5 minutes (they should remain crisp). Chill beans in cold water and drain.
2. Prepare vinaigrette.
3. Toss beans and mushrooms with vinaigrette and garnish with tomato slices.

Piquant Dijon Vinaigrette

1 clove garlic, finely chopped
2 shallots, finely chopped
3 tablespoons red wine vinegar
2 tablespoons olive oil
2 tablespoons water
1 tablespoon Dijon mustard
salt and pepper

1. Mix all ingredients in separate bowl. Add salt and pepper to taste.

Per serving: Calories—121   Fat—7 gms   Protein—3 gms
Carbohydrates—13 gms   Fiber—5 gms   Sodium—108 mgs

ROTINI WITH SQUEAKY CHEESE

Pasta and Company, Seattle

Deemed the "quintessential pasta salad of the '90s," this is Pasta and Co.'s best seller. Texture makes this dish exciting — the "squeaky" sensation of dry curd cottage cheese in the mouth. It features Quark, a spreadable cheese that may be substituted for sour cream or yogurt. Quark is available in either low- or nonfat versions at many grocery stores.

MAKES 11 CUPS

2 cups dry curd cottage cheese
1/3 cup plus 2 tablespoons nonfat Quark
1/3 cup plus 2 tablespoons white wine vinegar
2 tablespoons extra virgin olive oil
1 1/2 tablespoons fresh garlic, finely minced
1 1/2 teaspoons salt
cracked pepper to taste
2/3 pound fresh rotini pasta
1 1/2 cups green onions, thinly sliced
1 cup seeded unpeeled cucumber, cut in 1/4" cubes
16 cherry tomatoes, quartered
1/4 cup white wine vinegar
pinch of salt
2 tablespoons parsley, chopped

1. In a large bowl, fold together 1 1/2 cups cottage cheese (reserve remaining 1/2 cup), Quark, vinegar, olive oil, garlic, salt and pepper to taste.
2. Cook rotini in boiling, salted water. Rinse with cold water, drain well and fold into cottage cheese. Cool.
3. In a small bowl, toss tomatoes with vinegar and salt. Set aside. This can be done ahead of time — the longer the tomatoes soak the better the flavor.

SALADS & VEGETABLES

4. Fold green onions and cucumber in with the cooled pasta mixture.

5. Put pasta in a large serving dish. Top with tomatoes. Sprinkle with remaining cottage cheese and parsley. Serve at room temperature.

Per cup: Calories—107   Fat—3 gms   Protein—7 gms
Carbohydrates—13 gms   Fiber—1 gm   Sodium—332 mgs

TABOULI

Tabouli is a traditional middle Eastern salad made from bulgur wheat - wheat that has been pre-cooked, cracked and dried. Since it needs no further cooking, it's quick to prepare and ideal for summer days.

SERVES 3

1 cup bulgur wheat (tabouli)
1 cup cold water or reduced-fat chicken or vegetable broth
3 teaspoons olive oil
$\frac{1}{2}$ cup fresh parsley, chopped
2 tablespoons fresh mint, basil or cilantro, chopped
1 tablespoon lemon juice
1 clove garlic, crushed or minced
1 large tomato, chopped
$\frac{1}{2}$ avocado, diced
$\frac{1}{2}$ cucumber, diced (optional)
6 radishes, diced (optional)

1. Mix tabouli with water and oil. Refrigerate 1 hour to absorb water.

2. Before serving, mix in remaining ingredients.

Per serving: Calories—281   Fat—10 gms   Protein—8 gms
Carbohydrates—44 gms   Fiber—11 gms   Sodium—28 mgs

SPINACH SALAD

A special dressing makes this spinach salad stand out from the crowd. In summer, add fresh strawberries for an extra treat.

SERVES 4

2 bunches of spinach, about 4 cups
Poppyseed Balsamic Vinaigrette (recipe follows)
2 tablespoons green onion, chopped (garnish)

1. Wash and tear spinach into bite-size pieces. Put into large salad bowl.
2. Prepare vinaigrette and pour over spinach.
3. Toss salad and top with onions.

POPPYSEED BALSAMIC VINAIGRETTE

1 tablespoon poppyseeds
1 tablespoon sesame seeds
2 tablespoons sugar
$\frac{1}{4}$ cup balsamic vinegar
2 tablespoons olive oil
3 tablespoons grape or apple juice (grape adds nice flavor)
$\frac{1}{2}$ teaspoon Worcestershire sauce
$\frac{1}{2}$ teaspoon paprika

Mix all ingredients together.

Per serving: Calories—143   Fat—9 gms   Protein—3 gms
Carbohydrates—15 gms   Fiber—2 gms   Sodium—55 mgs

WALDORF SALAD

This recipe is a healthy update on a classic. By eliminating most of the fat, the salad is an excellent source of fiber, vitamins and minerals.

SERVES 6 TO 8

2 Red or Yellow Delicious apples, chopped
2 Fuji or Granny Smith apples, chopped
2 stalks celery, chopped
1 cup red or green seedless grapes
1/2 cup walnuts, chopped
1/2 cup raisins
salad greens
Waldorf Dressing (recipe follows)

1. Combine all salad ingredients.
2. In a separate bowl, mix all dressing ingredients.
3. Toss dressing with salad. Chill.
4. Serve on a bed of greens.

WALDORF DRESSING

3/4 cup plain nonfat yogurt
1/4 cup low-fat sour cream
1/4 cup low-fat mayonnaise
1/4 cup fresh orange juice
1/4 teaspoon ground nutmeg

Per serving: Calories—205   Fat—8 gms   Protein—5 gms
Carbohydrates—32 gms   Fiber—3 gms   Sodium—80 mgs

YUKON GOLD POTATO SALAD

Chef Jim Watkins, Plenty Cafe and Fine Foods, Seattle

A potato salad that is not only lightly dressed, but includes a medley of colorful vegetables. The addition of Provolone cheese provides that special flavor.

SERVES 8

2 sprigs rosemary
2 pounds Yukon Gold potatoes
salt and pepper to taste
1/4 cup olive oil
Dijon Vinaigrette (recipe follows)
6 ounces low-fat Italian Provolone, cut into bite-size chunks
2 medium zucchini, diced
5 Roma tomatoes, diced
1 yellow bell pepper, diced
1 green bell pepper, diced
1 bunch parsley, finely chopped
1 teaspoon celery seed

1. Preheat oven to 400° F.
2. Strip rosemary sprigs and chop fine. Slice potatoes in wedges and toss with rosemary, salt, pepper and olive oil. Bake for 15 minutes. Potatoes should still be firm enough for mixing.
3. Prepare vinaigrette and toss with potatoes.
4. Toss cheese, vegetables, parsley and celery seed with potatoes until thoroughly combined.
5. Serve in a large bowl or platter.

DIJON VINAIGRETTE

1/3 cup white wine vinegar
1 tablespoon Dijon mustard
1 teaspoon salt
1 teaspoon pepper
1/4 cup olive oil

Combine vinegar, mustard, salt and pepper in a blender. With blender running, add olive oil in a slow steady stream and process until emulsified.

Per serving: Calories—292   Fat—18 gms   Protein—8 gms
Carbohydrates—23 gms   Fiber—2 gms   Sodium—511 mgs

GARBANZO BEAN SALAD

A simple, healthy salad you can enjoy any time.

SERVES 2

4 leaves Romaine lettuce, cut into bite-size pieces
1 8-ounce can garbanzo beans, drained and rinsed
1/2 apple, chopped into small cubes
1/2 red or yellow bell pepper, cut into small cubes
Basic Nonfat Vinaigrette (see page 136)

1. Place vegetables and beans in salad bowl and toss with vinaigrette.

Per serving: Calories—227   Fat—3 gms   Protein—11 gms
Carbohydrates—40 gms   Fiber—7 gms   Sodium—14 mgs

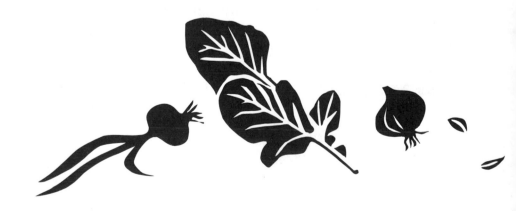

BROCCOLI AND TOFU

This is delicious hot or cold.

SERVES 4

4 stalks broccoli
1 red onion, sliced
1 red or yellow bell pepper, sliced thin
Marinated Tofu (recipe follows), prepared ahead
$\frac{1}{2}$ teaspoon sesame seeds

1. Trim and peel broccoli stems and cut into 2" pieces.
2. Steam broccoli stems and florets until slightly crunchy, about 5 minutes. Cool.
3. Toss onions and peppers together with broccoli.
4. Add Marinated Tofu and sprinkle with sesame seeds.

MARINATED TOFU

1 pound firm tofu, cut into $\frac{1}{2}$" pieces
3 garlic cloves, minced
$\frac{1}{2}$ cup balsamic vinegar
$\frac{1}{4}$ cup low-sodium soy sauce
1 tablespoon sesame oil
1 tablespoon fresh ginger, grated

1. Mix all ingredients except tofu in shallow bowl.
2. Add tofu and stir.
3. Refrigerate at least 30 minutes.
4. If you prefer to serve this dish hot, heat tofu in micro-wave for 2 minutes.

Per serving: Calories—217 Fat—10 gms Protein—15 gms
Carbohydrates—23 gms Fiber—7 gms Sodium—658 mgs

Tomato & Zucchini Gratin

Chef Jacques, of Queen Anne Thriftway and KIRO-TV.

A nice blending of flavors and textures that complements fish or poultry.

Serves 4

1 tablespoon olive oil
2 cloves garlic, crushed
2 tablespoons onion, chopped
2 sprigs basil, chopped
1/2 cup rice, uncooked
3/4 cup water
2 small zucchini, sliced 1/4" thick
4 medium tomatoes, sliced 1/2" thick
salt and pepper to taste
1/2 cup grated Asiago cheese, or 1/4 cup Parmesan or Romano
   (these are sharper than Asiago, so using less still gives
   ample flavor)

1. Preheat oven to 375° F.
2. Heat olive oil in a gratin dish or oven-proof skillet. Sprinkle garlic, onion and basil on top. Add rice and water.
3. Layer zucchini and tomato slices over rice. Add salt and pepper to taste. Bake for 20 minutes.
4. Sprinkle cheese on top and broil until golden brown. Serve at once.

Per serving: Calories—198   Fat—8 gms   Protein—7 gms
Carbohydrates—26 gms   Fiber—2 gms   Sodium—50 mgs

Vegetable Stir-Fry

Chef Jacques, of Queen Anne Thriftway and KIRO-TV, Seattle

A stir-fry with interesting flavors which can be varied with your choice of vegetable combinations. Using prepackaged stir-fry veggies is a real time and energy saver. Tofu may be added for extra protein. Accompany with jasmine rice or Oriental noodles.

SERVES 2

1 tablespoon peanut oil
1 teaspoon ginger, chopped
1 teaspoon garlic, chopped
package fresh stir-fry vegetables of your choice
1 tablespoon low-sodium soy sauce
1 tablespoon black bean sauce
1 teaspoon chili sauce
1/4 cup vegetable stock or water
1 teaspoon cornstarch
2 to 3 tablespoons water
1 teaspoon sesame oil

1. Heat peanut oil in a wok or skillet. Add ginger and garlic and stir-fry for 30 seconds. Add vegetables, soy, black bean and chili sauces and vegetable stock. Stir-fry for 3 minutes.
2. Mix cornstarch with water. Add cornstarch and sesame oil to stir fry. Give one final stir.

Per serving: Calories—186   Fat—9 gms   Protein—6 gms
Carbohydrates—22 gms   Fiber—7 gms   Sodium—759 mgs

SUMMER ROLLS WITH RED CHILI DIPPING SAUCE

Chef Alvin Binyua, Ponti Seafood Grill, Seattle

These delightful, vegetable-filled rolls may be served warm or at room temperature, steamed or not, accompanied by a lively homemade red chili sauce.

SERVES 6

1 tablespoon peanut oil
2 teaspoons garlic, minced
2 teaspoons fresh ginger, minced
1 cup carrots, cut into matchsticks
1 cup zucchini, cut into matchsticks
1 cup snow peas, cut into matchsticks
1 cup bean sprouts
1/4 cup basil leaves, thinly sliced
3/4 cup peanuts, chopped
24 sheets of rice paper (Bohn Trang)
pickled ginger (garnish)
Red Chili Sauce (recipe follows)

1. Pour oil into a hot frying pan. Fry garlic and ginger. Add other vegetables, stir-frying until crunchy, for about 30 seconds. Remove from heat, add peanuts if desired and set aside.
2. Soften each rice paper by dipping in lukewarm water. Put about 2 tablespoons vegetable mixture in the middle of each sheet. Fold sides over and roll each sheet up tightly. Serve as is with pickled ginger and Red Chili Sauce for dipping, or steam first as follows.
3. Place spring rolls in a bamboo steamer lined with parchment. Steam for 1 minute. Lift out carefully, as the rolls break easily. Lay on flat surface and cover with towel. Let sit 1 to 2 minutes before serving with pickled ginger and Red Chili Sauce.

RED CHILI-PEANUT DIPPING SAUCE

This spicy recipe makes about 2 cups.

1 cup water
3 teaspoons fish sauce
1 tablespoon red chili-garlic paste
1/4 cup brown sugar, packed
1 tablespoon cornstarch in 1/4 cup cold water
juice of 1/2 lime
2 tablespoons peanuts, chopped
1 tablespoon carrot, grated
2 teaspoons fresh basil, chopped

1. Bring water, fish sauce, chili-garlic paste and sugar to boil in saucepan.
2. Add cornstarch and simmer gently for 3 to 4 minutes. Remove from heat and cool.
3. Stir lime juice, peanuts, carrot and basil into cooled mixture.

Per serving: Calories—205   Fat—8 gms   Protein—5 gms
Carbohydrates—32 gms   Fiber—3 gms   Sodium—80 mgs

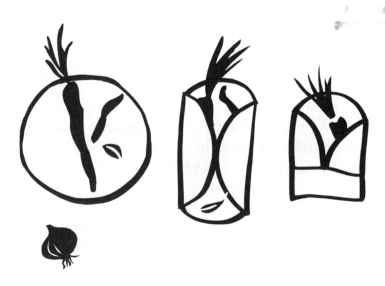

Cooking Whole Grains:
Brown Rice, Millet, Quinoa and Buckwheat

Onion, garlic or other chopped vegetables may be added to the grains before cooking. Seaweed, an excellent source of calcium, can also be added. (For dishes that cook longer than an hour, just cut the seaweed into small pieces and toss it in. For dishes that cook less than an hour, soak the seaweed for 10 minutes until it is soft enough to cut, then cut it up and throw it in.) For consistent quality, consider using a rice cooker.

Brown Rice ✓
Serves 2 to 3

1 cup short- or long-grain brown rice (a combination of white and brown rice may be used)
2 cups cold water (1 cup low-fat chicken or vegetable broth may be substituted for 1 cup water)
pinch of sea salt

1. Rinse rice and drain in a strainer.
2. In a covered saucepan, bring rice, water and salt to a boil. Reduce heat and simmer for an hour.

Per serving: Calories—342   Fat—3 gms   Protein—7 gms
Carbohydrates—71 gms   Fiber—3 gms   Sodium—118 mgs

Millet ✓
Serves 2 to 3

1 cup millet
3 cups water
pinch of sea salt

1. For a fluffier result, dry-roast millet in a skillet by stirring over medium heat until it smells toasty (optional).

2. Add millet and salt to boiling water. Turn down heat, cover and simmer for 25 minutes.

Per serving: Calories—378   Fat—4 gms   Protein—11 gms
Carbohydrates—-73 gms   Fiber—6 gms   Sodium—120 mgs

QUINOA ✓
(pronounced *keen-wah*)

SERVES 2 TO 3

1 cup quinoa
2¼ cups water
pinch of sea salt

Salt the water and bring it to a boil Add quinoa and turn down heat. Cover and let simmer 20 minutes.

Per serving: Calories—318   Fat—5 gms   Protein—11 gms
Carbohydrates—59 gms   Fiber—5 gm   Sodium—131 mg

BUCKWHEAT ✓
SERVES 2 TO 3

1 cup raw buckwheat (not roasted groats)
2 cups water

1. Dry-roast buckwheat in a skillet by stirring over medium heat until brown.
2. Bring water to boil. Add buckwheat and salt, turn down heat, cover and simmer for 20 minutes.

Per serving: Calories—292   Fat—3 gms   Protein—11 gms
Carbohydrates—61 gms   Fiber—9 gms   Sodium—8 mgs

OVEN FRIED POTATOES ✓

These potatoes are literally guilt-free. Sweet potatoes may also be fixed this way, or try a combination of white and sweet potatoes.

SERVES 6

6 cups potatoes (4 medium-size potatoes), peeled and diced
  into ½" cubes
1 cup onion, chopped
4 cloves garlic, chopped
3 tablespoons olive oil
2 tablespoons dried oregano
3 tablespoons toasted sesame seeds
3 tablespoons Parmesan cheese
1 teaspoon salt

1. Preheat oven to 425° F.
2. Arrange potatoes, onion and garlic on a nonstick cookie sheet.
3. Sprinkle potatoes with olive oil, oregano, sesame seeds,
Parmesan cheese and salt.
4. Bake for 45 minutes or until golden brown, turning every 15
minutes or so.

Per serving: Calories—196 Fat—10 gms Protein—4 gms
Carbohydrates—24 gms Fiber—2 gms Sodium—420 mgs

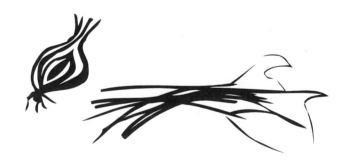

POLENTA WITH OPTIONS

Polenta is a tradition in Italian cuisine. This corn porridge can be made on top of the stove in less than 15 minutes. The consistency may vary from dense and firm to soft and creamy. The texture softens with longer cooking. It can be a quick and satisfying meal when combined with cheese and served with vegetables, beans or a salad. Or it can be served as a side dish with either meat, poultry or fish. If refrigerated, polenta keeps 3 to 5 days. To reheat, cut into squares and pop into the microwave or sauté in Sun-Dried Tomato Sauce (see page 140).

SERVES 4

2 cups low-sodium chicken broth
1½ cups water
1¼ cups polenta (coarse cornmeal)
Optional Additions:
¼ cup part-skim mozzarella, ricotta or Parmesan cheese
1 fresh tomato, sliced
1 clove fresh garlic, diced
½ teaspoon basil

1. Pour broth and water into a medium-size pan.
2. Add polenta and bring to a boil, whisking constantly.
3. Cook over medium heat, stirring frequently, for about 5 minutes or until thick and smooth.
4. Stir in options of your choice and remove from heat.

Per serving: Calories—205   Fat—3 gms   Protein—8 gms
Carbohydrates—36 gms   Fiber—4 gms   Sodium—80 mgs

POT BOILED RICE

For more flavor and extra fiber, minerals and protein, try adding other grains. Rye or wheat berries, dried corn, sweet brown rice, barley, lentils, kombu seaweed pieces or wild rice will all work well. Simply pre-soak ¼ cup of any selected grain for several hours, or bring grain to a boil in a covered pan for 5 minutes and set aside for an hour. Then add the grain to the 1 cup of rice and pot boil as instructed below.

SERVES 4

1 cup brown rice, short or long grain
2 cups water, or 1 cup low-sodium chicken broth and 1 cup water
pinch of sea salt
For larger batches, use less water proportionately
3 cups rice
5½ cups water

1. Rinse the rice and let drain.
2. Bring salted water to a boil in a medium-sized pan. Add the rice and any chosen grains, cover and turn the heat down to simmer. Cook for 50 to 60 minutes undisturbed.

Per serving: Calories—171 Fat—1 gm Protein—4 gms
Carbohydrates—36 gms Fiber—2 gms Sodium—111 mgs

Quinoa Topped with Glazed Shallots

Pasta and Company, Seattle

Care must be taken in preparing quinoa so it is not overcooked. Unique in texture, quinoa is extremely versatile. This dish is delicious served hot or at room temperature, and it reheats nicely.

SERVES 9

3/4 cup freshly squeezed lemon juice
1/2 cup vegetable or chicken stock
1/4 cup fresh garlic, coarsely chopped
1 teaspoon salt
1 teaspoon Tabasco
1/8 teaspoon ground cloves
1 pound uncooked quinoa
8 cups cold water
2 tablespoons olive oil
30 large shallots, peeled and sliced lengthwise
1 teaspoon sugar
2 tablespoons fresh parsley, finely chopped

1. In a large bowl, whisk together lemon juice, stock, garlic, salt, Tabasco and cloves. Set aside.
2. Pour uncooked quinoa into a bowl of cold water. Swirl it around and rinse through a fine mesh strainer. Complete this process three times or until water runs clear. Drain well.
3. Fill a saucepan with 8 cups cold water and add quinoa. Bring to a boil over high heat, stirring occasionally. Reduce heat and simmer for about 5 minutes. Quinoa should be partly translucent and slightly crunchy (not as soft as cooked cereal). Drain but do not rinse.

4. Spread quinoa out on a shallow-rimmed baking sheet, fluffing it with a fork. Fold in the dressing.

5. Heat olive oil in a sauté pan until nearly smoking. Add shallots and toss until they begin to brown.

6. Lower heat and add sugar. Allow shallots to cook very slowly until glazed and golden brown, 10 to 20 minutes.

7. Spoon quinoa into a serving bowl. Top with shallots, pan juices and parsley.

Per serving: Calories—281   Fat—6 gms   Protein—9 gms
Carbohydrates—50 gms   Fiber—4 gms   Sodium—310 mgs

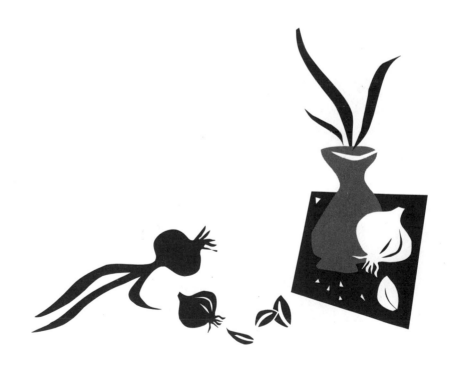

Quinoa Pilaf

The addition of sautéed onion, toasted sunflower seeds
or sesame seeds lend variety.

Serves 4

1 cup quinoa
2¼ cups water, boiling
pinch sea salt
1 tablespoon sautéed onion, or toasted sunflower or sesame seeds

1. To cook, roast quinoa in a skillet, stirring until golden. Add to boiling water, cover and simmer 20 minutes.
2. Stir in onion and/or sunflower or sesame seeds.

Per serving: Calories—160   Fat—2 gms   Protein—6 gms
Carbohydrates—30 gms   Fiber—3 gms   Sodium—161 mgs

POTATO PANCAKES

Recipes for potato pancakes vary only slightly, reflecting regional tastes. This variation includes leeks and garlic. Serve with apple-sauce or low-fat sour cream. Potato pancakes make a fine accompaniment for meat, poultry or fish.

SERVES 3

1 large russet potato, peeled and grated
½ cup leeks, chopped (may substitute onion)
2 tablespoons flour
¼ teaspoon salt
½ clove garlic, chopped
2 egg whites, beaten
olive oil

1. Preheat oven to 450° F.
2. Combine all ingredients except egg whites and oil and stir.
3. Fold in egg whites.
4. Dot a baking sheet with ½ teaspoon olive oil and drop a table-spoon of batter onto oil. Repeat until all batter has been used. Space pancakes 1" apart.
5. Bake for 15 minutes or until golden brown. Turn pancakes over and cook for another 10 minutes.

Per serving: Calories—84   Fat—1 gm   Protein—4 gms
Carbohydrates—15 gms   Fiber—1 gm   Sodium—220 mgs

RICE WITH LENTILS

This is a hearty one-pot dish.

SERVES 2

2 cups water
1½ cups reduced-fat chicken broth
1 small onion
2 cloves garlic, diced
2 carrots, sliced
¼ teaspoon white pepper
½ teaspoon ground cumin
½ cup lentils, washed
½ cup brown rice

1. In a large pan, combine all ingredients except lentils and rice. Bring to a boil.
2. When water is boiling, slowly stir in rice and lentils and return to boil.
3. Cover and reduce heat to low. Cook 45 minutes or until lentils and rice are tender.

Per serving: Calories—400   Fat—3 gms   Protein—20 gms
Carbohydrates—76 gms   Fiber—10 gms   Sodium—1155 mgs

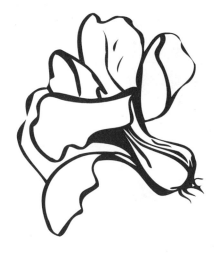

How to Prepare Beans

to reduce gas and bloating

1. Soak beans overnight. If time is short, use the double boil method described below.
2. Discard the soaking water and add fresh water.
3. Bring water to a boil and reduce heat. Simmer uncovered for 10 minutes. Skim off any foam. (Pressure-cooking big beans makes them extra tender.)
5. Consider adding kombu seaweed, a natural tenderizer.
6. Wait until the last 10 minutes to add salt.

"Double Boil" Method

This approach may be used for all types of beans except soy beans and garbanzo beans, which require soaking.

1. Pour beans into boiling water.
2. Bring water back to a boil.
3. Remove from heat.
4. Discard water and repeat the process.
5. Simmer beans until soft.

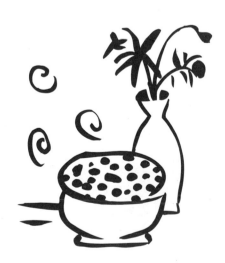

BEAN DIP ✓

This dip lends an appeal to raw vegetables that is truly irresistible. The dip also goes well with whole-grain crackers or low-fat baked tortilla chips.

MAKES ABOUT 2 CUPS

1 15-ounce can nonfat refried beans
$1/2$ teaspoon cumin
$1/3$ cup salsa
Optional:
  fresh tomatoes
  cilantro
  green chilies

Thoroughly mix all ingredients.

Per recipe: Calories—351   Fat—2 gms   Protein—20 gms
Carbohydrates—66 gms   Fiber—16 gms   Sodium—2079 mgs

BLACK BEANS

These distinctly flavored beans are an essential staple in Latin American cuisine.

SERVES 6

2 cups uncooked black beans, rinsed and cleaned
1 bay leaf
1/4 teaspoon dried oregano
1 teaspoon sugar
1 medium onion, chopped
2 cloves garlic, chopped
red or green bell pepper, chopped (optional)
1 teaspoon olive oil
chopped tomato, cilantro and green onions (optional garnish)

1. Place beans in a large bowl and cover with water. Soak overnight or for at least 6 hours.
2. Discard soaking water. Put beans in a large pot with bay leaf, oregano and sugar.
3. Add fresh water to cover and bring to a boil. Reduce heat and cook for about 2 hours or until beans are tender.
4. Using a nonstick skillet, sauté onion, garlic and bell pepper in olive oil for about 1 minute or until just opaque.
5. Add to cooked beans and simmer for 30 minutes to blend flavors.
6. Serve hot with rice and/or salsa. Garnish with tomato, cilantro or onion if preferred.

Per serving: Calories—227   Fat—2 gms   Protein—14 gms
Carbohydrates—40 gms   Fiber—14 gms   Sodium—2 mgs

GINGERED BLACK BEANS

An Asian adaptation of a South American favorite. Pinto, black-eyed or white beans may be substituted for the black turtle beans. This dish tastes even better the next day.

SERVES 6

1½ cups black turtle beans
4 cups water
1 strip kombu (seaweed)
2 teaspoons low-sodium soy sauce
1 teaspoon fresh ginger, finely grated

1. Rinse the beans, soak overnight and drain.
2. Bring water to a boil. Stir in beans, kombu, soy sauce and ginger. Reduce heat. Simmer 2 to 3 hours or until tender. Add water as needed to make enough sauce.

Per serving: Calories—158   Fat—0 gms   Protein—10 gms
Carbohydrates—30 gms   Fiber—7 gms   Sodium—81 mgs

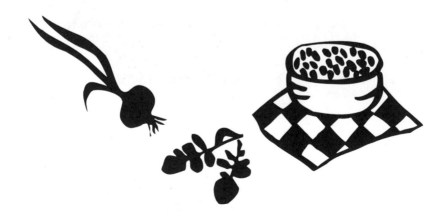

MEXICAN EGG AND BEAN CASSEROLE

Eggs that literally shout Olé! This dish is also known as chilaquiles.

SERVES 6

12 uncooked corn or wheat tortillas (if using frozen tortillas, be sure they are defrosted)
2 4-ounce cans diced green chilies
1 cup grated part-skim mozzarella or low-fat Jack cheese
1 15-ounce can nonfat refried beans
4 large eggs
2 cups buttermilk
cumin to taste

1. Preheat oven to 375° F.
2. Lightly grease a 2-quart casserole or a 9 x 13" pan.
3. Rip 6 tortillas into bite-size pieces and spread them evenly in pan.
4. Distribute 1 can chilies and ½ cup cheese over tortilla pieces. Spoon on beans in large dollops.
5. Tear remaining tortillas and spread them on top. Follow with remaining chilies and cheese.
6. Beat eggs and buttermilk together with cumin and slowly pour over casserole.
7. Bake for 30 minutes.

Per serving: Calories—375 Fat—9 gms Protein—22 gms
Carbohydrates—53 gms Fiber—10 gms Sodium—575 mgs

POLENTA AND BEAN CASSEROLE

A quick, wholesome and complete protein casserole that includes whole grains, beans and garlic. For a complete meal, serve with a tossed green or fruit salad.

SERVES 4

2 cups plus 2 tablespoons low-sodium chicken broth
1 cup polenta (coarse cornmeal)
$^1/_3$ cup part-skim mozzarella
1 whole chicken breast, skinned and boned, cut into 1" cubes
$^1/_2$ cup onion, chopped
2 cloves garlic, minced or pressed
$^1/_2$ teaspoon ground cumin
$^1/_2$ cup salsa
1 15-ounce can low-sodium beans, such as black, white, black-eyed or kidney

1. Preheat oven to 350° F.
2. Combine 2 cups broth and polenta in a medium-size pan. Bring to a boil, stirring constantly until thick and smooth, about 5 minutes.
3. Remove from heat. Stir in cheese and allow polenta to cool.
4. Cook chicken in 2 tablespoons broth for about 10 minutes or until chicken is white all the way through.
5. Add onion and garlic and cook until softened.
6. Add cumin and salsa.
7. Rinse beans in a colander to remove excess salt. Add to chicken.
8. Spread cooled polenta in the bottom of a nonstick 9 x 13 x 2" baking dish.
9. Spoon chicken and beans over polenta.
10. Bake for 20 minutes.

Per serving: Calories—356 Fat—5 gms Protein—28 gms
Carbohydrates—49 gms Fiber—7 gms Sodium—647 mgs

QUICK WHITE BEAN CHILI

A great and satisfying chili with a twist—it uses white beans.

SERVES 5 TO 7

3 cups boiling water
1/2 teaspoon chicken bouillon (dry powder or paste)
3 cloves garlic, chopped
1 medium onion, chopped
2 cups skinless chicken breast, diced
1 7-ounce can chopped green chilies
2 teaspoons ground cumin
1 teaspoon dried oregano
3/4 teaspoon cayenne
3 15-ounce cans low-sodium white beans
1/4 cup nonfat plain yogurt
3/4 cup low-fat sour cream
1 cup reduced fat Cheddar cheese, grated
avocado, chopped (optional)
parsley, chopped (optional)

1. Dissolve bouillon in boiling water.
2. Cook garlic and onion in 2 tablespoons of the bouillon
until soft.
3. Add chicken along with another 2 tablespoons broth and cook
until chicken is white all the way through.
4. Add chilies and spices, then beans and remaining broth.
Mix well.
5. Blend in yogurt, sour cream and cheese.
6. Heat thoroughly, stirring to avoid sticking.
7. Garnish with avocado and parsley, if desired.

Per serving: Calories—370   Fat—8 gms   Protein—30 gms
Carbohydrates—46 gms   Fiber—10 gms   Sodium—164 mg

VEGETARIAN CHILI

This hearty stew chili may also be served on a bed of rice, and corn bread makes a perfect accompaniment. For extra protein, cut firm tofu into $1/2$" cubes and add right before the chilies.

SERVES 6

2 tablespoons olive oil
$1/2$ cup onion, chopped
4 cloves garlic, minced
1 green bell pepper, diced
1 zucchini, diced
2 tablespoons chili powder
1 teaspoon ground cumin seed
1 teaspoon dry oregano
1 15-ounce can low-sodium pinto beans
1 15-ounce can low-sodium black beans
1 8-ounce can low-sodium garbanzo beans
1 15-ounce can tomato sauce
hot chilies to taste
grated cheddar cheese

1. Heat olive oil in a Dutch oven or saucepan. Sauté onion, garlic, green bell pepper and zucchini for 5 minutes.
2. Add remaining ingredients. Simmer for 30 minutes to combine flavors. Season with hot chilies to taste.
3. Serve in bowls with a sprinkling of grated cheddar cheese.

Per serving: Calories—338   Fat—7 gms   Protein—17 gms
Carbohydrates—55 gms   Fiber—17 gms   Sodium—500 mgs

Salad Dressing Hints

For nutritious salads, use low-fat dressings. Top carefully selected greens with the freshest ingredients.

A squeeze of lemon juice, a splash of wine or balsamic vinegar, or a drizzle of fruit juice can add just the right finishing touch to any salad.

Top with a selection of grated Parmesan cheese, garbanzo beans, raisins or aromatic herbs such as basil, marjoram, oregano, thyme, rosemary, chives or scallions.

Citrus Marinade

A sensational, semisweet marinade that includes garlic and citrus. It enhances the flavor of beef, chicken, fish or vegetables.

MAKES 2½ CUPS

$\frac{1}{3}$ cup lime juice
1 tablespoon lemon juice
$\frac{1}{3}$ cup low-sodium soy sauce
2 tablespoons Worcestershire sauce
1 tablespoon Grand Marnier (plum wine, sugar or sherry may be substituted)
1 cup orange juice, preferably freshly squeezed
4 to 5 cloves garlic, pressed
$\frac{1}{2}$ cup fresh cilantro, chopped
1" ginger, freshly grated (optional)

1. Mix all ingredients together.
2. Set meat in a shallow dish and pour marinade over it. Turn meat to coat all sides. Refrigerate at least 2 hours.
3. Grill, broil or stir-fry the meat.

Per recipe: Calories—266 Fat—1 gm Protein—9 gms
Carbohydrates—55 gms Fiber—1 gm Sodium—3446 mgs

Basic Nonfat Vinaigrette Dressing

A great basic dressing you can dress up as you like. Prepared in small amounts, it keeps well when stored in an airtight container in the refrigerator. Balsamic vinegar is used because it is less tart than other vinegars.

Makes 1 cup

½ cup balsamic vinegar
¼ cup apple or grape juice
3 tablespoons water
2 cloves garlic, minced
1 teaspoon lemon juice
¼ teaspoon Dijon mustard
Optional:
   ¼ teaspoon dried basil or thyme
   ¼ teaspoon dried oregano
   1 tablespoon toasted sesame seeds

1. Combine all ingredients in a small bowl.
2. Whisk until smooth.

Per tablespoon: Calories—13   Fat—0 gms   Protein—0 gms
Carbohydrates—2.5 gms   Fiber—0 gms   Sodium—4 mgs

Variation

To make a creamy vinaigrette, add 2 tablespoons nonfat yogurt.

Blue Cheese Vinaigrette

Combine ½ cup chopped walnuts and ½ cup diced blue cheese and sprinkle lightly over top of dressed greens.

Adds 3.5 fat grams

COOL AS A CUCUMBER

A simple recipe for <u>salad dressing</u> or <u>vegetable dip</u> that is low in fat but high in protein. It includes <u>fresh garlic</u> and nonfat <u>yogurt</u>, which are on the Top 10 "Super Foods" list. The <u>walnuts</u> are a good source of monounsaturated oils (see page 27 for details). Several variations on the basic recipe follow. Consider filling <u>pita bread</u> with <u>fresh vegetables</u>, and drizzling the dressing over the top.

MAKES ABOUT 2½ CUPS

1½ cups plain nonfat yogurt with live cultures (see note)
½ cup low-fat sour cream
2 cloves garlic, crushed
2 tablespoons lemon juice
2 tablespoons fresh dill, chopped
½ medium-size cucumber, grated very thin
¼ cup walnuts, chopped

Blend together all ingredients in a medium-size mixing bowl. Keep refrigerated until ready to serve.

Note: Yogurt can often be consumed by people who are lactose intolerant. Because yogurt with active cultures is predigested, the amount of milk sugars is very low.

Per tablespoon: Calories—15 Fat—1 gm Protein—1 gm
Carbohydrates—1 gm Fiber—0 gms Sodium—8 mgs

OLIVE OIL AND HERBS SPREAD

As a healthy alternative to butter, margarine or even "Better than Butter," try keeping the following mixture in your freezer as a handy and tasty spread for bread.

MAKES ABOUT 1/2 CUP

1/2 cup olive oil
1 tablespoon dried or 2 tablespoons fresh of your choice of basil, oregano, rosemary, red pepper flakes or garlic

1. Mix olive oil with other ingredients of your choice.
2. Pour into a cruet and place in freezer.
3. Store in freezer between uses.

Per tablespoon: Calories—120 Fat—14 gms Protein—0 gms
Carbohydrates—0 gms Fiber—0 gms Sodium—0 mgs

ZESTY NONFAT TOMATO DRESSING

A delicious alternative to traditional vinaigrettes.

MAKES 1 CUP

1/2 cup tomato juice
1 tablespoon lemon juice
1 tablespoon vinegar
1/4 teaspoon dry mustard or 1 teaspoon Dijon mustard
1 tablespoon finely chopped onion
1 teaspoon finely chopped parsley

1. Combine all ingredients.
2. Mix until well blended.

Per tablespoon: Calories—2 Fat—0 gms Protein—0 gms
Carbohydrates—1 gm Fiber—0 gms Sodium—36 mgs

BETTER THAN BUTTER

Butter is a natural whole food that is full of flavor and is a good source of vitamin A. By combining it with oil, water and buttermilk, you're taking an excellent step toward reducing your fat intake. Any quality vegetable oil may be used, but canola oil is recommended because it is monounsaturated. "Better than Butter" is great for baking or spreading on bread. It's so spreadable that it goes a long way.

MAKES 1 POUND

1 cup sweet cream butter
1 cup canola oil
1 cup buttermilk
1 cup ice water

1. Soften butter at room temperature.
2. Combine softened butter and oil in a deep bowl and mix until smooth.
3. Slowly add buttermilk and blend. Then add ice water and blend.
4. Store in refrigerator. "Better than Butter" will firm up when cooled. It also freezes well.

Per tablespoon: Calories—57 Fat—6 gms Protein—0 gms
Carbohydrates—0 gms Fiber—0 gms Sodium—33 mgs

Sun-Dried Tomato Sauce

This full-bodied, richly flavored tomato sauce complements a wide variety of dishes, including fish, tofu, vegetables and pizza - its versatility is virtually limitless. You'll definitely want to make extra to keep on hand because you'll love the convenience of flavorful dishes prepared in half the time.

MAKES 2 CUPS

1 cup boiling water
1 cup sun-dried tomatoes
3 large cloves garlic
1/4 cup fresh basil
4 teaspoons fresh parsley
1 tablespoon shallots
1 tablespoon lemon juice
1 tablespoon red wine vinegar
1 teaspoon Dijon mustard
1 teaspoon low-sodium soy sauce
2 tablespoons extra light olive oil
1/4 teaspoon salt
1/4 teaspoon red pepper flakes

1. Pour boiling water over sun-dried tomatoes and garlic. Soak 20 minutes.
2. Blend basil, parsley and shallots in the food processor until very fine.
3. Add softened tomatoes, garlic and 1/2 cup soaking liquid. Blend thoroughly.
4. Add lemon juice, vinegar, mustard, soy sauce, olive oil, salt and red pepper flakes. Blend until spreading consistency, adding extra soaking liquid if needed.

Per tablespoon: Calories—27   Fat—2 gms   Protein—1 gm
Carbohydrates—2 gms   Fiber—0 gms   Sodium—126 mgs

FETTUCCINE ORIENTAL

Chef Jacques, of Queen Anne Thriftway and KIRO-TV, Seattle

A pasta recipe that offers a delightful blending of exotic spices.

SERVES 4

4 medium shiitake mushrooms, thinly sliced
12 snow peas
1 pound fresh fettuccine
1 green onion, minced
Oriental Sauce (recipe follows)

1. Prepare Oriental Sauce.
2. Cook Oriental Sauce and mushrooms in a skillet over high heat for 3 minutes until sauce starts to thicken. Add snow peas and simmer for another minute.
3. While sauce is cooking, cook fettuccine in boiling, salted water for 2 minutes or until "al dente"—cooked firm to the bite.
4. Drain pasta and toss with sauce. Serve at once sprinkled with green onions.

ORIENTAL SAUCE

$\frac{1}{2}$ cup evaporated nonfat milk
$\frac{1}{4}$ cup dry sherry
1 teaspoon Hoisin sauce
1 tablespoon sesame oil
$\frac{1}{2}$ tablespoon fresh ginger, minced
$\frac{1}{2}$ tablespoon Chinese chili sauce

Combine all ingredients.

Per serving: Calories—411   Fat—6 gms   Protein—16 gms
Carbohydrates—70 gms   Fiber—5 gms   Sodium—141 mgs

FETTUCCINE WITH LOW-FAT ALFREDO

This quick and easy recipe calls for ricotta cheese that has been thinned with a little milk. Fresh Parmesan adds the final touch.

SERVES 5

1 pound whole-wheat fettuccine or linguine (or use a combination of whole wheat and white)
1 pound part-skim ricotta cheese
6 tablespoons nonfat milk
$1/3$ cup freshly grated Parmesan cheese
1 to 2 tablespoons "Better than Butter"
$1/2$ cup parsley, finely minced and well packed
salt and freshly ground black pepper to taste

1. Cook pasta in boiling, salted water for about 2 minutes or until "al dente"—cooked firm to the bite. Drain.
2. Beat ricotta and milk in large bowl until creamy and smooth. Stir in $1/4$ cup Parmesan which may be preheated in microwave for 1 minute.
3. Immediately stir cheese sauce into cooked pasta and blend in "Better than Butter."
4. Add parsley. Salt to taste. Grind black pepper over top and sprinkle with remaining Parmesan.

Per serving: Calories—497 Fat—12 gms Protein—27 gms
Carbohydrates—74 gms Fiber—9 gms Sodium—266 mgs

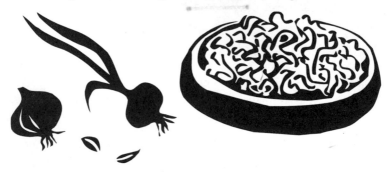

142

LASAGNA

*Tofu boosts the protein content of this hearty vegetarian dish
without changing the traditional flavor. Other vegetables such as
broccoli, chard or precooked eggplant may be used. Low-fat
cottage cheese may be substituted for all or part of the tofu or
ricotta cheese.*

SERVES 12

1 recipe Basic Spaghetti Sauce (see page 144)
1 cup soft tofu
2 cups low-fat ricotta cheese
½ cup part-skim mozzarella cheese, grated or shredded provolone
¼ cup Parmesan cheese, grated
9 cooked lasagna noodles (combination of white and whole-grain
   may be used)
1 10-ounce package frozen chopped spinach, thawed and drained
2 zucchini, sliced

1. Preheat oven to 350° F.
2. Combine tofu, ricotta, mozzarella and 2 tablespoons of
Parmesan in a bowl and mix well.
3. Spread a thin layer of sauce in the bottom of a 9 x 13 x 2"
baking pan.
4. Arrange a layer of noodles on top. They may touch but should
not overlap. Cover them with half the vegetables, half the cheese
mixture and ⅓ of the sauce.
5. Repeat with another layer of noodles, vegetables, cheese and
sauce.
6. Arrange remaining noodles on top. Cover with remaining sauce.
Sprinkle with mozzarella and remaining 2 tablespoons Parmesan.
7. Bake for 45 minutes or until bubbly and vegetables are tender.
8. The lasagna may be frozen either before or after cooking. Allow
for extra baking time if frozen.

Per serving: Calories—263   Fat—9 gms   Protein—14 gms
Carbohydrates—34 gms   Fiber—5 gms   Sodium—897 mgs

Basic Spaghetti Sauce

A versatile red sauce that can either serve as a topping for pizza or be served over pasta or rice. It keeps in the refrigerator for up to a week, or may be frozen. The flavor of the sauce will vary depending upon the ingredients chosen.

SERVES 6 TO 8

1 onion, chopped
1 red bell pepper, chopped
1 green bell pepper, chopped
2 large carrots, chopped
3 cloves garlic, minced
3 tablespoons olive oil
2 28-ounce cans tomato purée
1 tablespoon low-sodium soy sauce
1 tablespoon sweetener (sugar or honey)
1 teaspoon salt
1 teaspoon oregano
1 teaspoon marjoram
$\frac{1}{2}$ teaspoon pepper
$\frac{1}{2}$ teaspoon thyme
1 bay leaf

In a large pot, sauté onion, bell peppers and garlic in olive oil until soft. Add remaining ingredients. Simmer for an hour, stirring occasionally.

Per serving: Calories—181   Fat—6 gms   Protein—5 gms
Carbohydrates—31 gms   Fiber—7 gms   Sodium—1307 mg

Pasta Provençale au Gratin

Chef Jacques, of Queen Anne Thriftway and KIRO-TV, Seattle

The full, fresh flavor of tomatoes and basil is further enhanced by the addition of Parmesan cheese.

Serves 6

3 cups elbow macaroni
3 medium tomatoes, peeled and coarsely chopped
1/2 cup fresh basil, chopped
2 tablespoons olive oil
1/2 cup Parmesan cheese, grated
salt and pepper to taste

1. Preheat oven to 400° F.
2. Cook pasta in a large pot of boiling salted water for about 10 minutes. Drain well and place in a large bowl. Add tomatoes, basil, olive oil and half the Parmesan cheese. Mix well. Season with salt and pepper.
3. Transfer mixture to a 9 x 13" baking dish. Top with remaining Parmesan. Bake for about 10 minutes or until brown. Serve at once.

Per serving: Calories—281   Fat—8 gms   Protein—11 gms
Carbohydrates—41 gms   Fiber—3 gms   Sodium—162 mgs

PIZZA

A delightful Sunday night treat that's bursting with flavor. Olives, zucchini, onions, tomatoes, anchovies, capers or hot peppers may be added to suit individual tastes, and it can be made without cheese for those who are lactose intolerant. The unraised dough freezes well.

MAKES TWO 12" PIZZA CRUSTS

CRUST

1 cup lukewarm water or milk
1 package active dry yeast
$\frac{1}{2}$ teaspoon salt
1 tablespoon olive oil
2 cups all-purpose unbleached flour
$\frac{1}{2}$ cup whole-wheat pastry flour
cornmeal

SUGGESTED TOPPINGS

2 cups tomato purée
4 tablespoons Sun-Dried Tomato Sauce (see page 140)
4 ounces grated part-skim mozzarella
4 ounces part-skim ricotta cheese
8 cloves garlic, thinly sliced
crushed red pepper
$\frac{1}{4}$ teaspoon oregano
1 green bell pepper, sliced into thin rings
$\frac{1}{4}$ pound mushrooms, thinly sliced

1. Preheat oven to 500 degrees F.
2. Pour lukewarm water into a medium-size bowl and sprinkle in yeast. Let stand 5 minutes until foamy.
3. Add salt, olive oil and $\frac{1}{2}$ cup flour. Beat for several minutes with a wooden spoon.
4. Add remaining flour, $\frac{1}{2}$ cup at a time, mixing by hand after

146

each addition. The dough should be a bit softer than bread dough but not as sticky.

5. Turn dough out onto a surface lightly dusted with cornmeal and knead for 5 minutes. Clean and oil mixing bowl before returning the dough. Place the bowl in a warm place (an unheated oven works well) for ½ to ¾ hour or until dough has risen and doubled in bulk.

6. Oil two 12" pizza pans, or divide dough in half and freeze for later use. Allow 3 hours to thaw.

7. Punch dough down, return it to dusted surface and knead for several minutes.

8. Halve dough and roll out to fit pans. Put it in the pan and press into place. Brush top lightly with olive oil. Spread tomato purée and tomato sauce over dough. Cover with cheeses and toppings.

9. Bake pizza on top oven rack for 10 to 12 minutes or until crust is golden and toppings are bubbling. Serve immediately.

Per slice: Calories—257   Fat—7 gms   Protein—12 gms
Carbohydrates—40 gms   Fiber—4 gms   Sodium—511 mgs

MACARONI AND CHEESE

A quarter of the fat has been cut from this traditional favorite.

SERVES 4

1 7-ounce box Macaroni and Cheese
1 cup whole-grain elbow macaroni
2 tablespoons "Better than Butter"
⅓ cup nonfat milk

1. Boil boxed macaroni with extra cup macaroni.
2. Use "Better than Butter" instead of butter.
3. Moisten ingredients with milk.
4. Mix in cheese packet and serve.

Per serving: Calories—280   Fat—6 gms   Protein—11 gms
Carbohydrates—50 gms   Fiber—6 gms   Sodium—249 mgs

A TWO-STEP PIZZA

An Italian dish that is easy to prepare yet achieves a sensational pizza-like result. Makes great leftovers.

SERVES 8

CRUST

1 cup polenta (coarse cornmeal)
1½ cups low-sodium chicken broth
1½ cups water
½ teaspoon salt
2 egg whites, beaten

1. Combine polenta, broth, water and salt in a saucepan. Bring to a boil and simmer for about 10 minutes, stirring frequently until thick.
2. Remove from heat and blend in egg whites.
3. Lightly grease a 9" pie pan. Form the polenta into a thick crust in pan. Let stand.

TOPPING

½ cup onions, diced
½ cup green bell peppers, diced
½ cup red bell peppers, diced
1 clove garlic, crushed
½ cup diced tomatoes
1 teaspoon oregano
1 tablespoon olive oil
1 cup low-fat mozzarella, grated

1. Preheat oven to 350° F.
2. Sauté onions, bell peppers and garlic in olive oil until tender. Remove from heat and stir in tomatoes and oregano.
3. Spread onto the polenta crust. Cover with grated cheese. Bake for 45 minutes.

Per serving: Calories—140 Fat—5 gms Protein—8 gms
Carbohydrates—17 gms Fiber—2 gms Sodium—239 mgs

BRAISED PORK CHOPS

Braising is a slow cooking method that tenderizes tougher and leaner cuts of meat, allowing rich flavors to develop. Meat and vegetables are browned in a Dutch oven in a small amount of broth, water or other nonfat liquid. The stock is then added and the meat is simmered until tender. Rice, mashed potatoes, noodles or polenta make fine accompaniments.

SERVES 4

4 6-ounce boneless pork chops, trimmed of fat
2 tablespoons all-purpose unbleached flour
3 tablespoons chicken broth
1 small onion, diced
$\frac{1}{2}$ cup mushrooms, sliced
2 cups low-sodium chicken broth (may substitute nonfat milk)

1. Coat pork chops with flour. In a nonstick skillet, brown chops in 3 tablespoons chicken broth.
2. Move chops to one side, add onion and mushrooms. Sauté for 1 minute.
3. Return pork chops to middle of pan, add 2 cups broth or milk and cover. Simmer for 30 minutes or until tender, stirring occasionally.
4. Remove chops from pan and stir sauce. If a thicker sauce is desired, make a paste of 1 tablespoon each of water and flour and stir into sauce until thickened. Serve chops and sauce separately.

Per serving: Calories—306 Fat—13 gms Protein—40 gms
Carbohydrates—5 gms Fiber—0 gms Sodium—138 mgs

FAJITAS

These tasty fajitas call for marinated flank steak, but you can substitute boned and skinless chicken, fish fillets or a 10-ounce package of silken, firm-style light or reduced-fat tofu. As another alternative, try half tofu and half beef, chicken or fish. Serve fajitas with nonfat refried beans, rice or our Black and White Bean Salad (see page 103).

SERVES 6

12-ounce flank steak, cut into 1" strips and marinated in Citrus
    Marinade (see page 135) for at least 30 minutes
1 medium onion, sliced
1 green bell pepper, sliced in long, narrow strips
1 red bell pepper, sliced in long, narrow strips
3 cloves garlic, diced
6 flour tortillas
2 tomatoes, chopped
salsa (optional)
cilantro, minced (optional)
avocado, chopped (optional)
plain nonfat yogurt or low-fat sour cream (optional)

1. Heat a nonstick skillet or wok. Stir-fry steak strips for 5 to 8 minutes.
2. Add vegetables and stir-fry until just tender.
3. Heat tortillas. Fill each tortilla with an equal measure of meat and vegetables. Garnish with your choice of tomato, salsa, cilantro, avocado, plain low-fat yogurt or low-fat sour cream.

Per serving: Calories—308   Fat—9 gms   Protein—18 gms
Carbohydrates—39 gms   Fiber—3 gms   Sodium—428 mgs

MEAT LOAF

A new twist on an all-American favorite. Substituting ground chicken breast for half the meat helps to significantly reduce the fat content. Steamed vegetables such as potatoes, carrots, turnips or rutabagas make a fine accompaniment.

SERVES 6

1 pound lean ground beef
1 pound ground chicken breast (or substitute
   10 ounce package tofu)
1 medium onion, chopped
2 cloves garlic, diced
1 medium carrot, coarsely grated
$\frac{1}{2}$ cup oats, quick cooking or regular
2 eggs
1 7.5-ounce can low-sodium stewed tomatoes
$\frac{1}{8}$ teaspoon pepper (optional)

1. Preheat oven to 350° F.
2. Mix ground beef and chicken or tofu in a large bowl with onion, garlic, carrot, oats and eggs.
3. Chop or blend tomatoes. Season with pepper and combine with chicken.
4. Shape into loaf and place in a loaf pan.
5. Cover and bake for 60 minutes. Uncover and brown for about 15 minutes. Make sure the meat is well done.

Per serving: Calories—334 Fat—16 gms Protein—36 gms
Carbohydrates—10 gms Fiber—2 gms Sodium—131 mgs

LAMB STIR-FRY WITH BROCCOLI

Serve with jasmine rice or Oriental noodles.

SERVES 4

Garlic-Ginger Marinade (recipe follows)
1 pound leg of lamb or loin meat, cut into thin strips
Soy-Sherry Sauce (recipe follows)
2 cups broccoli flowerettes
2 tablespoons peanut oil
2 cloves garlic, minced
1 tablespoon cornstarch
2 to 3 tablespoons water

1. Prepare marinade, add lamb and refrigerate for 20 minutes.
2. Prepare sauce and set aside.
3. Blanch broccoli in salted, boiling water for 2 minutes. Cool in cold water. Drain and set aside.
4. Heat 1 tablespoon oil in a wok. Stir-fry lamb for 1 minute. Return meat to marinade.
5. Heat remaining oil in the wok. Stir-fry garlic with broccoli for 30 seconds. Add lamb and pour in sauce. Bring to a boil. If desired, thicken sauce with cornstarch mixed with water.

GARLIC-GINGER MARINADE

2 tablespoons oyster sauce
2 tablespoons low-sodium soy sauce
2 tablespoons cornstarch
1 tablespoon dry sherry
2 cloves garlic, minced
1 tablespoon fresh ginger, minced

Mix all ingredients in bowl.

Soy-Sherry Sauce

¼ cup chicken stock
2 tablespoons low-sodium soy sauce
2 tablespoons sherry vinegar
1 teaspoon sesame oil
1 teaspoon Chinese chili sauce
1 tablespoon cilantro, minced

Mix all ingredients together well.

Per serving: Calories—352   Fat—24 gms   Protein—21 gms
Carbohydrates—12 gms   Fiber—1 gm   Sodium—1067 mgs

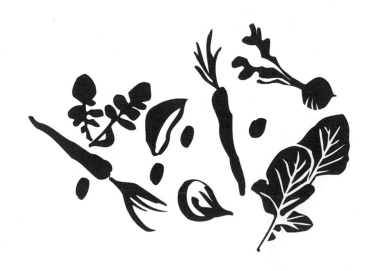

Roasted Chicken

This full-flavored chicken is easy to prepare. Consider rubbing fresh basil, oregano, thyme, sage or cilantro under the skin, or adding a quartered orange along with the garlic and onion in the body cavity to enhance the flavor even more.

Serves 4 to 6

3 to 4 pound whole frying or roasting chicken
1 small onion, peeled and cut in half
2 cloves garlic
1 teaspoon poultry seasoning
1 teaspoon curry powder (optional)
$\frac{1}{2}$ cup water or chicken broth

1. Preheat oven to 400° F.
2. Remove giblets and neck from body cavity. Rinse chicken well and pat dry with a paper towel.
3. Fill bird cavity with onion and garlic. Place chicken breast side up in a roasting pan.
4. Sprinkle seasonings over chicken and rub them in well.
5. Add water or chicken broth.
6. Cover and cook for $\frac{1}{2}$ hour. Baste with pan drippings, adding more water or broth as necessary to keep bird moist. Cook another hour, basting as needed. Uncover to brown the last 15 minutes.
7. Remove skin before eating. The skin of a chicken contains a large amount of fat. Removing the skin before eating reduces the total fat intake from 47 grams to 10 grams of fat per serving.

Per serving: Calories—387   Fat—10 gms   Protein—68 gms
Carbohydrates—2 gms   Fiber—0 gms   Sodium—246 mgs

EASY CHICKEN DIVAN

*Here is a quick and easy low-fat revision of a
familiar chicken casserole.*

SERVES 6

1 10-ounce package frozen broccoli (or fresh), partially cooked
1 to 1½ cups sliced cooked skinless chicken breast
1 can Special Request Cream of Chicken soup (not diluted)
½ cup light mayonnaise
1 teaspoon lemon juice
¼ teaspoon curry powder
¼ cup shredded low-fat Cheddar cheese
½ cup soft bread crumbs

1. Preheat oven to 350° F.
2. Arrange cooked broccoli in greased 11 x 7" baking casserole.
Place chicken on top.
3. Combine soup, mayonnaise, lemon juice and curry powder and
pour over chicken. Sprinkle with cheese and bread crumbs.
4. Bake for 25 to 30 minutes, or until thoroughly heated.

Per serving: Calories—119   Fat—6 gms   Protein—8 gms
Carbohydrates—8 gms   Fiber—1 gm   Sodium—224 mgs

CHICKEN BISCUIT PIE

Although this recipe looks complicated, it really isn't—and it's a complete and satisfying meal. Leftover chicken or turkey may be substituted for the chicken breasts.

SERVES 8

Biscuit Topping (recipe follows)
3 cups skinless, boneless chicken breasts, diced
2 15-ounce cans low-sodium chicken broth
1 medium red potato, unpeeled and diced
1 stalk celery, chopped
$\frac{1}{2}$ cup red bell pepper, chopped
2 cloves garlic, minced
2 medium carrots, thinly sliced
1 small leek, chopped
1 cup fresh mushrooms, sliced
1 small can "petite pois" peas
$\frac{1}{4}$ cup white flour
2 tablespoons whole-wheat pastry flour
$\frac{1}{2}$ teaspoon poultry seasoning
$\frac{1}{4}$ teaspoon pepper
1 cup skim milk

1. Preheat oven to 400° F.
2. Prepare biscuit dough but do not bake.
3. In a nonstick skillet, cook chicken in $\frac{1}{4}$ cup broth for 10 minutes or until done. Set aside.
4. In a large saucepan over medium-high heat, bring chicken broth to a boil. Add potato, celery, red bell pepper and garlic. Cover and cook 5 minutes. Add carrot and leek and simmer 3 minutes. Add mushrooms and peas and cook 5 minutes, or until tender.
5. In a small bowl, combine flour, poultry seasoning and pepper. Whisk in milk. Pour into saucepan with vegetable mixture and cook over medium heat for 3 minutes until thickened and bubbly, stirring constantly. Remove from heat and add chicken.

MEAT, POULTRY, FISH & TOFU

6. Pour chicken and vegetables into a nonstick 9 x 13 x 2" baking dish. Using a large tablespoon, place 16 spoonfuls of biscuit dough on top, spacing evenly. Bake for 28 minutes or until biscuits are golden brown.

BISCUIT TOPPING

1 cup white flour
1 cup whole-wheat pastry flour
2 teaspoons baking powder
$\frac{1}{2}$ teaspoon salt
1 cup nonfat milk or buttermilk
1$\frac{1}{2}$ tablespoons "Better than Butter," melted

1. Combine all dry ingredients and mix well.
2. Add milk and "Better than Butter" and stir just until moistened.

Per serving: Calories—304   Fat—7 gms   Protein—24 gms
Carbohydrates—35 gms   Fiber—3 gms   Sodium—412 mgs

CINNAMON ROASTED CHICKEN BREAST

Chef Ludger Szmania, of Szmania, Seattle

The bed of dressed seasonal greens provides an elegant presentation for this aromatic dish.

SERVES 8

4 7-ounce chicken breasts, skinned
Savory Cinnamon Marinade (recipe follows)
2 to 3 tablespoons olive oil
Garlic Vinaigrette (recipe follows)
¾ pound seasonal greens

1. Preheat oven to 350° F.
2. Place chicken in large pan.
3. Prepare marinade, pour over chicken and refrigerate overnight.
4. Remove chicken from marinade and pat dry.
5. Heat olive oil in large skillet over high heat. Sear chicken each side for 2 to 3 minutes, or until brown.
6. Transfer chicken with hot oil to ovenproof platter and bake for 10 minutes or until done.
7. Prepare vinaigrette and salad of seasonal greens.
8. Slice chicken and lay atop dressed seasonal greens.

SAVORY CINNAMON MARINADE

$1/2$ cup red wine vinegar
3 cups water
1 cup low-sodium soy sauce
3 tablespoons ground cinnamon
$1/2$ teaspoon nutmeg
$1/2$ teaspoon allspice
$1/2$ teaspoon ground cloves
pepper to taste

Combine all ingredients.

GARLIC VINAIGRETTE

6 cloves garlic, peeled
$1/2$ yellow onion
$1/2$ cup water
$1/3$ cup vinegar
$2/3$ cup water
fresh herbs, chopped
salt and pepper to taste
dash of sugar

1. In a small saucepan, boil garlic and onion in $1/2$ cup water until tender.
2. Put all ingredients in blender and process for 5 seconds.
3. Toss with seasonal greens.

Per serving: Calories—199   Fat—7 gms   Protein—25 gms
Carbohydrates—10 gms   Fiber—3 gms   Sodium—800 mgs

CHICKEN SATE WITH PEANUT SAUCE

Chef Jacques, of Queen Anne Thriftway and KIRO-TV, Seattle

Serve with jasmine rice and peanut sauce on the side.

SERVES 4

8 bamboo skewers soaked in water
2 cloves garlic, chopped
2 tablespoons low-sodium soy sauce
1 tablespoon ground turmeric
2 tablespoons lime juice
1 pound skinless, boneless chicken breasts, cut into $1/2$" pieces
16 fresh mushroom caps
1 cup any peanut sauce at room temperature

1. Preheat oven to Broil.
2. Combine garlic, soy sauce, turmeric and lime juice in a large bowl. Add chicken and toss until evenly coated. Refrigerate for 2 hours.
3. Remove chicken from marinade and thread onto skewers. Place 1 mushroom on end of each skewer.
4. Place skewers under broiler or on barbecue. Cook 5 to 8 minutes per side, or until crisp and brown.
5. Serve with peanut sauce for dipping.

Per serving: Calories—112   Fat—5 gms   Protein—2 gms
Carbohydrates—17 gms   Fiber—2 gms   Sodium—98 mgs

CITRUS CHICKEN WITH DIJON MUSTARD

Dijon mustard gives this dish its special tangy flavor.
Serve with rice or pasta.

SERVES 4

4 skinless, boneless chicken breasts
2 tablespoons Dijon mustard
1/2 cup onion, chopped
1/2 cup red bell pepper, chopped
4 cloves garlic, minced
1 tablespoon olive oil
1/4 cup orange juice
1 tablespoon lemon juice
2 tablespoons brown sugar

1. Coat chicken breasts on each side with Dijon mustard.
2. In a large skillet, lightly sauté onion, red bell pepper and garlic in olive oil. Put vegetables on a plate.
3. Place chicken in pan and brown on both sides. (Add a little more olive oil if needed.)
4. Add sautéed vegetables and reduce heat.
5. Mix orange and lemon juices with brown sugar. Pour over chicken and simmer, covered, for 1 hour or until very tender.

Per serving: Calories—229 Fat—7 gms Protein—28 gms
Carbohydrates—13 gms Fiber—1 gm Sodium—257 mgs

Roast Chicken with 40 Cloves of Garlic

Chef Jacques, of Queen Anne Thriftway and KIRO-TV, Seattle

A delightfully seasoned chicken with just a slight taste of garlic.

Serves 6

4 pound free-range or roasting chicken, skinned
40 cloves garlic, unpeeled
2 lemons
salt and pepper
1 tablespoon olive oil
2 shallots, peeled
8 to 12 small red potatoes, unpeeled

1. Preheat oven to 400° F.
2. Fill the chicken cavity with 10 crushed garlic cloves and 1 lemon, cut in half. Truss chicken and place in a shallow roasting pan. Season with salt and pepper. Drizzle olive oil and juice from remaining lemon over bird. Arrange potatoes in pan. Roast for 30 minutes.
3. Add shallots and remaining 30 cloves of garlic. Cook an additional 30 minutes or until chicken juices run clear.
4. Remove chicken, potatoes and garlic to a warm serving platter. Stir one cup of water into roasting pan. Scrape any drippings off pan bottom and simmer for 5 minutes. Strain and serve in a sauce boat.

Per serving: Calories—514   Fat—11 gms   Protein—66 gms
Carbohydrates—37 gms   Fiber—3 gms Sodium—237 mgs

ROSEMARY ROASTED CHICKEN

Chef Jacques, of Queen Anne Thriftway and KIRO-TV, Seattle

This chicken is delicious served either hot or cold.

SERVES 6

4 pound whole free-range or roasting chicken
salt and pepper
6 sprigs fresh rosemary
10 cloves garlic, unpeeled
8 to 12 small red potatoes
4 small onions or shallots, peeled
1 tablespoon olive oil
salt and pepper

1. Preheat oven to 400° F.
2. Place chicken in a shallow roasting pan. Season inside and out with salt and pepper. Fill bird's cavity with rosemary and 4 garlic cloves. Arrange potatoes around bird, drizzle with olive oil and place in oven.
3. After 30 minutes, add onions and remaining 6 garlic cloves. Cook another 30 minutes or until chicken juices run clear.
4. Remove skin before eating.

Per serving: Calories—524 Fat—12 gms Protein—68 gms
Carbohydrates—33 gms Fiber—3 gms Sodium—241 mgs

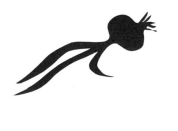

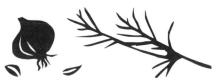

STIR-FRY SZECHUAN CHICKEN

Chef Jacques, of Queen Anne Thriftway and KIRO-TV, Seattle

A spicy entrée that can be quickly prepared.
Serve with jasmine rice or Oriental noodles.

SERVES 4

4 skinless, boneless chicken breasts, sliced into strips
3 tablespoons Hoisin sauce
1 tablespoon low-sodium soy sauce
2 tablespoons garlic, minced
2 tablespoons fresh ginger, minced
2 tablespoons cornstarch
Szechuan Sauce (recipe follows)
1 tablespoon peanut oil
$\frac{1}{2}$ tablespoon Szechuan peppercorns, crushed
1 small zucchini, cut in strips 3" long by $\frac{1}{4}$" wide
8 ears of canned baby corn
2 to 3 tablespoons water

1. In a bowl, combine chicken strips with Hoisin and soy sauces.
Add 1 tablespoon each of garlic, ginger and cornstarch. Marinate
for 20 minutes.
2. Prepare Szechuan Sauce.
3. Heat peanut oil in a wok and stir-fry chicken for 2 minutes.
Remove chicken from wok and set aside.
4. Heat remaining oil in wok and stir-fry 1 tablespoon each garlic
and ginger with Szechuan peppercorns for 20 seconds. Add zucchini, corn and Szechuan Sauce. Cook for 2 minutes. Add chicken.
Mix remaining tablespoon of cornstarch with water and stir into
sauce to thicken as desired.

Szechuan Sauce

1/4 cup dry sherry
1/2 tablespoon Chinese chili sauce
1 tablespoon sherry vinegar

Blend all ingredients.

Per serving: Calories—239   Fat—7 gms   Protein—29 gms
Carbohydrates—12 gms   Fiber—1 gm   Sodium—462 mgs

Salmon in Sun-Dried Tomato Sauce

A variation on a Pacific Northwest favorite, inspired by the Greeks.

Serves 4

4 5-ounce salmon fillets
4 tablespoons Sun-Dried Tomato Sauce (see page 140)

1. Preheat nonstick frying pan on medium-high heat.
2. Spoon tomato sauce into pan.
3. Place salmon on top, skin-side down.
4. Cook for 5 to 7 minutes or until brown. Turn fish over and continue cooking for another 5 minutes or until done.

Per serving: Calories—269   Fat—16 gms   Protein—29 gms
Carbohydrates—1 gm   Fiber—0 gms   Sodium—129 mgs

TORTILLA WRAPS WITH TROPICAL FRUIT SALSA

David deVarona, owner of Todo Loco Restaurants, Seattle

This is a great "portable feast." The ingredients for the fresh fruit salsa can vary according to your taste and what is in season.

SERVES 3

1 9-ounce chicken breast, skinned and boned
1 tablespoon honey
1 teaspoon ground cumin seed
3 whole-wheat tortillas
1½ cups jasmine rice, or any kind, cooked
6 tablespoons Tropical Salsa (recipe follows)
2 tablespoons prepared sweet chili sauce
9 to 12 fresh basil leaves

1. Rub chicken with honey and sprinkle with cumin and bake or broil for 10 – 15 minutes, or until done. Cut into strips.
2. Prepare Tropical Salsa.
3. Assemble by placing ½ cup rice in center of each tortilla and layer with 3 ounces chicken, 2 tablespoons salsa, 3 to 4 basil leaves and 2 teaspoons sweet chili sauce.
4. Wrap by folding up opposite sides about 1" to form the bottom and top. Roll up from one "side" to the other and serve. To make portable, just wrap in foil.

Tropical Salsa

1 fresh mango, peeled, pitted and diced
1 pint fresh strawberries, sliced
$\frac{1}{2}$ fresh pineapple, peeled and diced
juice of 1 lime
2 tablespoons chopped cilantro
1 serrano chili pepper, minced (optional)

Place all ingredients in small bowl and mix together well.

Per serving: Calories—639 Fat—8 gms Protein—35 gms
Carbohydrates—109 gms Fiber—5 gms Sodium—524 mgs

CIOPPINO

A zesty seafood stew that uses our Basic Spaghetti Sauce (see page 144) for its stock.

SERVES 4

2 cups Basic Spaghetti Sauce (see page 144)
$\frac{1}{2}$ cup water, apple juice, wine or chicken broth
fresh parsley, minced
basil, dill and cumin to taste
2 cups seafood of your choice, such as shrimp, clams, mussels
    and chunks of halibut, sole and salmon (salmon has a higher
    fat content than white fish)
cooked rice
Parmesan cheese, grated, for garnish

1. Heat sauce and liquid in large skillet. Add seasonings to taste.
2. Add seafood and simmer for 5 to 8 minutes, turning fish once.
Cook until fish is just done.
3. Serve over rice and top with a light sprinkling of Parmesan.

Per serving, using 1 cup each halibut and shrimp: Calories—271 Fat—7 gms
Protein—31 gms Carbohydrates—24 gms Fiber—5 gms Sodium—1147 mgs

Scallop and Vegetable Stir-Fry

This delightful combination of asparagus, mushrooms and scallops is sure to please.

Serves 4 to 6

3 tablespoons low-sodium soy sauce
1 teaspoon cornstarch
2 tablespoons sesame oil
6 asparagus spears, trimmed and cut into 1" pieces
6 mushrooms, sliced
3 green onions, sliced (1 medium leek may be substituted, but use only the white and green portion)
1 medium carrot, peeled and sliced
1/2 red bell pepper, cut into matchstick-size pieces
1 zucchini, sliced
3 large cloves garlic, finely chopped
2 teaspoons fresh ginger, minced
1/2 pound bay scallops, fresh or frozen

1. Combine soy sauce with cornstarch in a small dish.
2. Lightly coat a nonstick skillet or wok with sesame oil. Turn heat on high. Add asparagus, mushrooms, onions, carrot, red pepper, zucchini, garlic and ginger. Stir-fry about 8 minutes.
3. Add scallops and cook for 6 minutes, or until vegetables are tender and scallops are white throughout.
4. Stir in soy sauce and cook for 1 minute or until thickened. Serve immediately.

Per serving: Calories—128 Fat—6 gms Protein—10 gms
Carbohydrates—9 gms Fiber—2 gms Sodium—443 mgs

FETTUCCINE AND SCALLOPS

Chef Jacques, of Queen Anne Thriftway and KIRO-TV, Seattle

Serve with a tossed green salad and a crusty loaf of Italian bread.

SERVES 4

1 pound fresh spinach fettuccine
2 tablespoons olive oil
4 cloves garlic, minced
4 medium shiitake mushrooms, thinly sliced
½ pound bay scallops
½ cup tomatoes, diced
4 sprigs Italian parsley, minced
salt and pepper
½ cup Asiago, Parmesan or Romano cheese, grated

1. Heat olive oil in a large skillet. Stir in garlic and mushrooms.
Cook for 1 minute. Add scallops and stir vigorously for 1 minute.
Add tomatoes, parsley, and salt and pepper to taste.
2. Cook pasta in boiling, salted water for about 2 minutes or until
"al dente"—cooked firm to the bite.
3. Drain and toss with scallops. Top with freshly grated cheese.
Serve immediately.

Per serving: Calories—291   Fat—12 gms   Protein—18 gms
Carbohydrates—27 gms   Fiber—2 gms   Sodium—135 mgs

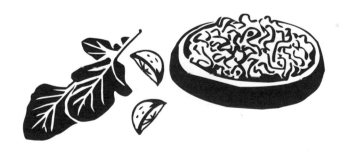

GINGER BAKED FISH

A delicious and easy way to prepare a variety of fish.

SERVES 2

$\frac{1}{2}$ teaspoon fresh ginger, grated
$\frac{1}{2}$ teaspoon low-sodium soy sauce
6 to 8 ounce fillet of sole, bass, halibut or red snapper
$\frac{1}{2}$ teaspoon toasted sesame oil

1. Preheat oven to 350° F.
2. Combine ginger and soy sauce.
3. Lightly baste both sides of the fish with sesame oil, then with ginger-soy sauce mixture.
4. Place fish in a nonstick baking pan. Bake for 15 to 20 minutes or until flaky and tender. Serve with a lemon wedge.

Per serving: Calories—104   Fat—2 gms   Protein—19 gms
Carbohydrates—1 gm   Fiber—0 gms   Sodium—230 mg

YOGURT AND DILL BAKED FISH

A delightful way to enhance the mild taste of cod or red snapper.
You can also use salmon, which has a higher fat content.

SERVES 4

4 6-ounce cod or red snapper fillets
2 teaspoons dried dill
$1\frac{1}{3}$ cups nonfat yogurt
4 lemon wedges

1. Preheat oven to 350° F.
2. Arrange fish on nonstick baking sheet.
3. Sprinkle each fillet with $\frac{1}{2}$ teaspoon dill and top each with $\frac{1}{3}$ cup yogurt.

4. Bake for 15 to 20 minutes or until fish begins to flake.
5. Serve with fresh lemon wedges.

Per serving, using cod: Calories—352 Fat—1 gm Protein—39 gms
Carbohydrates—6 gms Fiber—0 gms Sodium—142 mgs

POACHED FISH

Poaching is an easy way to bring out the delicate flavor of fresh fish. Salmon is an excellent source of omega-3 fatty acids – one of a group of essential fatty acids that have been shown to exert beneficial effects on the immune system.

SERVES 4

4 6-ounce salmon fillets, or any mild fish
2 cups white wine
4 celery tops
2 cloves garlic, chopped
1 onion, chopped
1 teaspoon dill weed

1. Put wine, celery tops, garlic and onion into a large, deep pot. Add enough water to cover fish.
2. Bring water to a boil on medium-high heat.
3. Sprinkle fish with dill and set into boiling water. (Hint: To prevent fish from falling apart when removing it from the bath, wrap it in cheesecloth before immersing.)
4. Cook 10 to 20 minutes, depending on thickness of fillets, or until done.

Note: Salmon is higher in fat than less fatty white fish, such as cod.

Per serving (using salmon): Calories—405 Fat—18 gms Protein—35 gms
Carbohydrates—4 gms Fiber—1 gm Sodium—117 mgs

Per serving (using cod): Calories—273 Fat—2 gms Protein—39 gms
Carbohydrates—5 gms Fiber—1 gm Sodium—140 mgs

ORANGE CRUSTED HALIBUT WITH SAUTÉED WATERMELON

Executive Chef Kerry Sear, Four Seasons Hotel, Seattle

An elegant, healthy entrée that is easily prepared.

SERVES 4

4 5-ounce halibut fillets
2 teaspoons olive oil
salt and pepper
$1/4$ cup orange zest (see note below)
1 cup bread crumbs
2 tablespoons parsley, chopped
2 tablespoons basil, chopped
$1/2$ cup white wine
$1/2$ cup orange juice
4 cups seedless watermelon, cut in 1" squares
1 cup white onion, peeled and chopped
1 pinch red chili pepper flakes
$1/2$ cup white wine
$1/2$ cup bell peppers, chopped

1. Preheat oven to 350° F.
2. Lightly rub halibut with olive oil and season with salt and pepper. Mix together orange zest, bread crumbs, parsley and basil. Coat each piece of halibut with this mixture.
3. Place in shallow dish with $1/2$ cup wine and orange juice and bake for 10 minutes. If bread crumbs start to get too dark, cover with foil.
4. Heat a skillet or wok over medium heat and add $1/2$ cup wine, onions and peppers. Cook until vegetables are soft.
5. Sprinkle in chili flakes and add watermelon. Stir constantly until watermelon mixture is warm.
6. Pour sauce onto 4 plates and place halibut on top.

MEAT, POULTRY, FISH & TOFU

Note: to make orange zest, grate just the colored outer part of the rind with a fine grater, or thinly peel it off the fruit with a vegetable peeler and chop in food processor. Do not include the white part of the rind.

Per serving: Calories—405 Fat—8 gms Protein—35 gms
Carbohydrates—40 gms Fiber—3 gms Sodium—301 mgs

HALIBUT WITH TOMATOES AND BASIL

Chef Jacques, of Queen Anne Thriftway and KIRO-TV, Seattle

Serve with rice.

SERVES 4

4 6-ounce halibut fillets
2 tablespoons olive oil
2 cloves garlic, minced
1 cup tomatoes, skinned and diced
juice of 1 lemon
$\frac{1}{2}$ cup basil leaves, chopped
salt and pepper

1. Heat olive oil in a skillet. Cook halibut for one minute on each side.
2. Add garlic, tomatoes, lemon juice and basil around the fillets. Simmer for two minutes. Add salt and pepper to taste.
3. Spoon sauce onto the bottom of each plate. Place fish on top and garnish with a sprig of fresh basil.

Per serving: Calories—263 Fat—11 gms Protein—36 gms
Carbohydrates—4 gms Fiber—1 gm Sodium—97 mgs

TOFU TACOS

Having extra "Sun-Dried Tomato Sauce" and "Cool as a Cucumber Dressing" on hand makes preparing these tacos a snap. Otherwise, the tofu can be sautéed in 2 teaspoons olive oil along with 1 clove chopped garlic and $1/4$ cup tomato sauce. Add $1/3$ cup low-fat yogurt combined with 1 clove pressed garlic, 1 tablespoon lemon juice and 1 teaspoon tahini sauce to the cabbage.

MAKES 2 TACOS

1 tablespoon Sun-Dried Tomato Sauce (see page 140)
$1/2$ 10-ounce package firm silken tofu (1% fat)
2 cups red cabbage, finely chopped
$1/3$ cup cilantro, chopped
$1/3$ cup Cool as a Cucumber dressing (see page 137)
2 whole-wheat tortillas or chapati bread

1. Sauté tofu in tomato sauce until lightly browned.
2. Mix cabbage, cilantro and cucumber dressing together.
3. Warm tortillas and fill with tofu and cabbage mixture.

Per taco: Calories—143   Fat—3 gms   Protein—9 gms
Carbohydrates—27 gms   Fiber—4 gms   Sodium—235 mgs

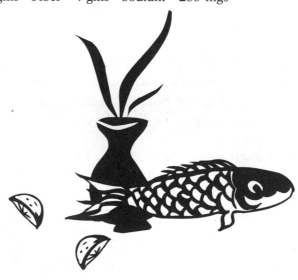

BAKED APPLES

A delicious way to end any meal.

SERVES 4

4 large baking apples
1/4 cup chopped pecans
1/4 cup raisins
1/4 to 1/2 cup honey
2 teaspoons "Better than Butter"

1. Preheat oven to 375° F.
2. Wash apples and remove cores to 1/2" of bottoms. Cut a strip of peel from around top of each apple.
3. Fill each apple with 1 tablespoon each pecans and raisins. Drizzle 1 to 2 tablespoons of honey over nuts and raisins and dab 1/2 teaspoon "Better than Butter" on top.
4. Place in 8 x 8" baking dish with 3/4 cup boiling water. Bake 40 to 60 minutes, until tender. Baste with pan juices and serve.

Per serving: Calories—257 Fat—7 gms Protein—1 gm
Carbohydrates—53 gms Fiber—5 gms Sodium—8 mgs

BERRIES AND YOGURT

A delicious way to take advantage of summer's bounty.

SERVES 4

1 quart fresh strawberries
1/2 cup powdered sugar
1 cup nonfat yogurt

1. Rinse and drain strawberries in a colander.
2. Arrange berries on a serving plate.
3. Set out a bowls of powdered sugar and yogurt for dipping.

Per serving: Calories—136 Fat—1 gm Protein—4 gms
Carbohydrates—30 gms Fiber—2 gms Sodium—48 mgs

BLACKBERRY UPSIDE-DOWN CAKE
WITH MOCK CRÈME FRAÎCHE

Chef Jim Watkins, Plenty Cafe and Fine Foods, Seattle

A light dessert that uses a slurry of flaxseed and water as an egg substitute. Look in the packaged grain and flour section of large supermarkets or health food stores for flaxseed. If it's unavailable, you can use 3 eggs or the equivalent in egg substitute.

SERVES 8

$\frac{1}{4}$ cup flaxseed
$\frac{3}{4}$ cup water
2 tablespoons "Better than Butter"
$\frac{1}{2}$ cup brown sugar
3 cups blackberries
pinch of salt
1$\frac{1}{2}$ teaspoons vanilla extract
1 teaspoon lemon zest
$\frac{1}{2}$ cup sifted all-purpose flour
Mock Crème Fraîche (recipe follows), prepared ahead

1. Preheat oven to 375° F.
2. To make slurry, process flaxseed in spice grinder or coffee grinder, pour into a blender and process with water until smooth.
3. In a cast-iron 9" skillet, melt butter with 3$\frac{1}{2}$ tablespoons brown sugar over moderate heat until bubbly, stirring constantly, about 3 minutes. Arrange blackberries in one layer in skillet and simmer over low heat, stirring gently, until they begin to give up their juices, about 10 minutes. Remove from heat.
4. Beat slurry with salt and remaining sugar in an electric mixer on high speed until mixture reaches 3 times its original volume, about 8 minutes.
5. Stir in vanilla and lemon zest. Sift flour over top and fold gently in.

6. Pour batter over berries. Bake for 20 minutes. Cool on a rack for 7 minutes before inverting onto a serving plate. Serve with a generous dollop of Mock Crème Fraîche.

Mock Crème Fraîche

¾ cup low-fat sour cream
¾ cup buttermilk

Whisk sour cream and buttermilk together. Cover bowl with plastic wrap and refrigerate overnight. Makes about 1½ cups.

Per serving: Calories—166   Fat—5 gms   Protein—3 gms
Carbohydrates—28 gms   Fiber—3 gms   Sodium—78 mgs

Simply Strawberry Shortcake

A delightful summertime favorite. Hint: Because this recipe doubles the size of the buttermilk biscuits, allow for extra baking time.

Serves 6

1 quart strawberries
1 recipe for Buttermilk Biscuits (see page 84)
3 tablespoons date sugar
low-fat vanilla frozen yogurt

1. Preheat oven to 375° F.
2. Add date sugar to dry biscuit ingredients.
3. Follow biscuit recipe instructions, but make 6 large biscuits instead of 12 smaller ones.
4. Bake for 15 minutes.
5. Allow biscuits to cool slightly.
6. Split biscuits while still warm. Spoon on freshly cut strawberries and top with frozen yogurt.

Per serving: Calories—271   Fat—7 gms   Protein—7 gms
Carbohydrates—47 gms   Fiber—5 gms   Sodium—706 mgs

BAKED CUSTARD

A smooth dessert to satisfy your sweet tooth.

SERVES 5

2 cups low-fat milk (2%)
1/4 to 1/3 cup honey
1/8 teaspoon salt
2 eggs
1 teaspoon vanilla
nutmeg to taste

1. Preheat oven to 325° F.
2. Warm milk with honey and salt, stirring until honey is dissolved.
3. Beat eggs lightly and slowly add warmed milk while stirring constantly.
4. Add vanilla.
5. Pour mixture into 5 custard cups that have been placed in a baking pan. Sprinkle with nutmeg. Pour hot water around cups to a depth of 1 inch.
6. Bake 45 to 60 minutes.
7. Custard is done when knife blade inserted in center comes out clean.

Per serving: Calories—142   Fat—4 gms   Protein—6 gms
Carbohydrates—22 gms   Fiber—0 gms   Sodium—126 mgs

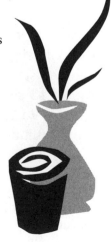

BERRY FRUIT CRISP

A delicious, summery dessert.

SERVES 6

3 cups fresh or frozen berries (raspberries and marionberries
  are especially good)
$2/_3$ cup all-purpose unbleached flour
2 tablespoons cornstarch
$1/_2$ cup oats, regular or quick cooking
$1/_2$ cup nuts, chopped, such as pecans, walnuts, almonds or
  hazelnuts
$1/_2$ cup brown sugar
1 teaspoon cinnamon
$1/_2$ teaspoon salt
$1/_2$ cup "Better than Butter"
vanilla-flavored low-fat frozen yogurt

1. Preheat oven to 350° F.
2. Combine berries in an 8" square baking pan.
3. Lightly spoon flour into a measuring cup.
4. Combine flour with remaining dry ingredients in a mixing
bowl. Work in "Better than Butter" by hand until consistency is
crumbly. Sprinkle over fruit.
5. Bake for 45 minutes or until golden brown and bubbly. Serve
warm, topped with frozen yogurt.

Per serving: Calories—326   Fat—15 gms   Protein—6 gms
Carbohydrates—44 gms   Fiber—4 gms   Sodium—230 mgs

CHOCOLATE CHIP COOKIES

These whole-grain cookies contain less fat and sugar than most cookies and make a nutritious snack.

MAKES 30 COOKIES

$\frac{1}{2}$ cup "Better than Butter"
$\frac{1}{4}$ cup date sugar
$\frac{1}{4}$ cup brown sugar
2 egg whites
$\frac{1}{2}$ teaspoon vanilla
$\frac{3}{4}$ cup whole-wheat pastry flour
$\frac{1}{4}$ cup plus 2 tablespoons oat flour
$\frac{1}{2}$ teaspoon salt
$\frac{1}{2}$ teaspoon baking soda
$\frac{1}{2}$ cup nuts, chopped (walnuts or pecans are best)
$\frac{1}{2}$ cup chocolate chips

1. Preheat oven to 375° F.
2. Blend "Better than Butter" and date and brown sugars together until creamy.
3. Beat in egg whites and vanilla.
4. Sift dry ingredients, then stir into mixture.
5. Stir in nuts and chocolate chips.
6. Drop dough by teaspoonfuls onto a nonstick cookie sheet, spacing them well apart.
7. Bake about 10 minutes.

Per cookie: Calories—71   Fat—4 gms   Protein—2 gms
Carbohydrates—9 gms   Fiber—1 gm   Sodium—70 mgs

CHOCOLATE CHIP MINT COOKIES

These whole-grain cookies are a lower fat, lower sugar variation on an old favorite. To make a chocolate chip orange cookie, simply substitute orange extract for the peppermint extract.

MAKES 24 TO 30 COOKIES

$^3/_4$ cup "Better than Butter"
$^3/_4$ cup date sugar
$^1/_4$ cup brown sugar
2 egg whites
1 teaspoon peppermint extract
1 teaspoon vanilla
$1^1/_2$ cups whole-wheat pastry flour
$^1/_4$ cup unsweetened cocoa
$^1/_4$ teaspoon salt
1 teaspoon baking soda
$^1/_2$ cup semisweet chocolate chips

1. Preheat oven to 350° F.
2. Blend "Better than Butter" with date and brown sugars until creamy.
3. Beat in egg whites, peppermint and vanilla.
4. Sift together dry ingredients and add with chocolate chips to butter mixture.
5. Drop dough by teaspoonfuls onto a nonstick cookie sheet, spacing them well apart.
6. Bake about 10 to 12 minutes.

Per cookie: Calories—112   Fat—5 gms   Protein—2 gms
Carbohydrates—17 gms   Fiber—2 gms   Sodium—98 mgs

OATMEAL CAKE

This dessert is rich in flavor, but minus the usual fat found in cake. If "Better than Butter" is not available, substitute ¼ cup oil combined with ¼ cup buttermilk.

SERVES 12

1 cup 3-minute oats
½ cup "Better than Butter"
1¼ cups boiling water
1 egg
2 egg whites
1 cup brown sugar
½ cup date sugar
1½ teaspoons vanilla
1 cup whole-wheat pastry flour
½ cup all-purpose unbleached flour
1 teaspoon baking soda
1 teaspoon cinnamon
¾ teaspoon ginger
½ teaspoon allspice
¼ teaspoon salt
¼ teaspoon cloves

1. Preheat oven to 350° F.
2. Combine oats, "Better than Butter" and boiling water in a bowl. Stir and set aside for about 15 minutes.
3. Beat eggs, sugar and vanilla together.
4. Sift dry ingredients.
5. Add oats to brown and date sugars and mix well.
6. Stir in dry ingredients.
7. Pour batter into a nonstick 9 x 13" baking pan. Bake for 25 to 30 minutes or until a knife inserted into the middle comes out clean. Sprinkle with powdered sugar.

Per serving: Calories—226   Fat—5 gms   Protein—4 gms
Carbohydrates—42 gms   Fiber—3 gms   Sodium—36 mgs

Pumpkin Pie

A low-fat creation that is truly deserving of special praise.

Serves 12

9 whole graham crackers
$\frac{1}{2}$ cup fruit juice
4 egg whites, whipped
1 16-ounce can pumpkin
$\frac{1}{2}$ cup brown sugar
$\frac{1}{4}$ teaspoon salt
1 teaspoon ground cinnamon
$\frac{1}{2}$ teaspoon ground ginger
$\frac{1}{4}$ teaspoon ground cloves
1 12-ounce can evaporated skim milk

1. Preheat oven to 425° F.
2. Finely crush graham crackers. Combine crumbs with fruit juice, just to moisten. Press into a 9" pie plate.
3. In a large mixing bowl, combine remaining ingredients in order listed. Blend until smooth.
4. Pour filling into prepared pie crust.
5. Bake for 15 minutes.
6. Reduce oven temperature to 350 degrees and bake an additional 40 to 50 minutes or until a knife inserted near the center comes out clean. Cool before serving.

Per serving: Calories—125   Fat—1 gm   Protein—4 gms
Carbohydrates—25 gms   Fiber—1 gm   Sodium—254 mgs

Rhubarb Coffee Cake

The tart flavor of rhubarb is an annual springtime treat. The date sugar used in this recipe can be found at many grocery stores.

Serves 12

½ cup "Better than Butter"
¾ cup date sugar
¾ cup brown sugar
1 egg
1 cup buttermilk
1 cup all-purpose unbleached flour
1 cup whole-wheat pastry flour
1 teaspoon baking soda
1 teaspoon vanilla
2 cups fresh rhubarb, finely chopped

Topping

½ cup sugar
1 teaspoon cinnamon

1. Preheat oven to 350° F.
2. Cream "Better Than Butter" with date and brown sugar in a large bowl.
3. Add egg and buttermilk. Beat until smooth.
4. Gradually add flour, baking soda and vanilla. Mix well.
5. Fold in rhubarb.
6. Pour into a 9 x 13" nonstick baking pan.
7. Mix topping and spread evenly over top of cake.
8. Bake for about 45 minutes.

Per serving: Calories—265 Fat—5 gms Protein—4 gms
Carbohydrates—53 gms Fiber—3 gms Sodium—162 mgs

Pears in Orange Sauce

A refreshing dessert that is easily prepared, yet special enough for company.

SERVES 2

1 tablespoon sugar
2 teaspoons lemon juice
$1/4$ cup orange juice
$1^1/_2$ teaspoons cornstarch
1 teaspoon grated orange peel
1 pear, cored and sliced into 6 wedges

1. In small saucepan, combine all ingredients except pear and cook over medium heat until thick, stirring constantly.
2. Arrange pear slices on serving plates. Pour sauce over pear and chill.

Per serving: Calories—97   Fat—0 gms   Protein—1 gm
Carbohydrates—25 gms   Fiber—2 gms   Sodium—1 mg

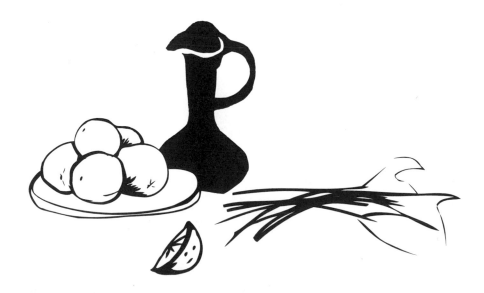

GLOSSARY

Antioxidants: Any of a variety of naturally occurring substances—such as vitamins A, E, and C; beta-carotene; and selenium—that can prevent or impede oxidation reactions.

Carcinogens: Cancer-causing substances.

Carotenoids: A class of plant pigments found in dark green and orange vegetables and fruits, that have proven antioxidant and immune-regulatory abilities.

Complete protein: Refers to a food that contains sufficient amounts of all eight essential amino acids that your body needs but can't produce on its own.

Complex carbohydrates: Refers to foods composed of long chains of linked sugar complexes (carbohydrates). Commonly used to refer to grains, breads, and starchy vegetables.

Cruciferous vegetables: A group of vegetables (including cauliflower, cabbage, brussels sprouts, broccoli, turnips, and rutabagas) containing substances that may protect against and fight cancer.

Enzymes: Protein-like substances, formed in plant and animal cells, that act as catalysts in initiating or speeding up specific chemical reactions. Usually destroyed by high temperatures.

Flavonoids: A group of plant pigments proven to protect against free-radical damage. Noted for their anti-inflammatory, antiviral, antiallergenic and anticancer activities.

Free radicals: Highly reactive compounds with at least one unpaired electron. Formed naturally within the body as a result of metabolic processes. The body is also exposed to free radicals as a result of sun exposure (radiation), smoking, drug and alcohol use, pollution, and stress. Free radicals can cause oxidative damage to cell membranes, tissue, and DNA and contribute to aging and disease progression, including cancer.

Incomplete protein: A food that is low in or lacks one or more of the eight essential amino acids. All plant foods, except soy, are incomplete proteins, but they can be combined with other plant foods containing the deficient amino acid(s) in sufficient amounts to form a complete protein. The combination of rice and beans is an example of a complete-protein meal.

Indoles: A group of compounds, found in cruciferous vegetables, that have exhibited anticancer activity.

Isoflavin/flavones: A group of compounds, found in soy and other plant foods, that may block the entry of estrogen into cells, reducing the risk of breast and ovarian cancer.

Lactose: A form of sugar found in milk and other dairy products.

Lactose intolerance: The inability to digest milk sugar (lactose) due to insufficient production of lactase, the enzyme that digests lactose. Lactase production typically declines with age, and may be reduced by certain diseases and disease treatments that cause changes to the small intestine.

Legumes: The protein-rich seeds of plants such as kidney beans, soybeans, garden peas, lentils, black-eyed peas, and lima beans. Legumes are a good source of soluble fiber and can exert a stabilizing effect on blood sugar levels.

Limonene: A phytochemical found in citrus fruits that may step up the production of enzymes that help dispose of potential carcinogens.

Macronutrients: Protein, carbohydrates, and fats are called *macronutrients* because the body needs them in large quantities.

Macrophage: A type of white blood cell that filters the lymph system, engulfing foreign particles such as bacteria and cellular debris.

Micronutrients: Vitamins and minerals are called micronutrients because the body needs them in small quantities.

Nitrosamines: Carcinogens formed during digestion from nitrites—food additives used to prevent bacterial growth in processed meats such as hot dogs, bacon, ham, and sausage. In adequate doses, vitamin C can prevent the transformation of nitrites to nitrosamines.

Omega-3 fatty acids: Fats found in cold-water fish, such as salmon, mackerel, and herring, and in certain plants and seeds, such as evening primrose, flax, and borage seeds. Omega-3 fatty acids have been shown to positively affect immune responses, reduce the inflammation response to injury and infection, decrease the formation of blood clots, lower blood pressure, and reduce cholesterol.

Phytochemicals: *Phyto* means plant. *Phytochemicals* is a generalized term for a wide group of naturally occurring substances, such as limonene, that are found in plants and have been shown to have anticancer effects.

Phytoestrogens: Phytoestrogens are natural substances, found in soy and other plant foods, that exert estrogen-like effects. Compared to estrogen, phytoestrogen's activity is only 1:400. Because of this weak effect, phytoestrogens tend to counteract extreme estrogen levels; if estrogen levels are low, they will cause an increase in estrogen effect; if levels are too high, phytoestrogens will bind to estrogen-binding sites, thus decreasing estrogen's effects. In men, phytoestrogens seem to block testosterone, the hormone that can spur the growth of prostate tumors.

Phytosterols: Substances—found in plants—that may slow the production of cells in the large intestine and therefore slow tumor growth.

Protease inhibitors: Compounds that inhibit the action of protein-digesting enzymes and may retard the growth of human colon and breast cancer cells.

Saponin: A sugar compound with emulsifying properties. Saponins are thought to interfere with the process by which DNA replicates, and they may prevent cancer cells from multiplying.

Selenium: A trace mineral and important antioxidant that may help prevent cancer formation and promotion. Selenium functions either alone or as part of enzyme systems. Although selenium is needed only in small amounts, insufficient intake is common because of selenium-deficient soils. Low-selenium diets have been associated with an increased risk of cancer.

Sulphoraphane: A sulfur-based chemical found in plants that may stimulate enzymes in the body to destroy cancer-causing agents.

Terpene: May decrease cholesterol and increase enzymes known to break down carcinogen.

REFERENCES

INTRODUCTION
Page 1

1. "It is generally accepted that 30 percent of all cancers are linked to diet."
American Institute for Cancer Research Information Series, revised Nov. 1991. *The Cancer Process.*

2. "What's more, what we eat may have a significant impact on..."
Nixon, D. W. 1994. *The Cancer Recovery Eating Plan.* New York: Times Books, Random House.

3. "The American Dietetic Association supports the use of nutrients..."
Quillin, P. 1994. *Beating Cancer with Nutrition.* Tulsa, Okla.: Nutrition Times Press, Inc.

4. "In 1980 the National Cancer Institute commissioned..."
National Research Council. *Diet, Nutrition, and Cancer.* Washington, D.C.: National Academy Press.

Making Healthier Food Choices
Page 4

1. "Many in the scientific community believe that 30 percent of all cancers..."
American Institute for Cancer Research Information Series, revised Nov. 1991. *The Cancer Process.*

2. "For the person with cancer, a healthy diet has been shown to make..."
Hamilton, E. N., E. N. Whitney, F. S. Sizer. 1991. *Nutrition Concepts and Controversies,* 5th Ed. Saint Paul, Minn.: West Publ. Co.

THE TOP 10 "SUPER FOODS"
Cruciferous Vegetables
Page 6

1. "In a University of Minnesota study in the 1970s..."
Wattenberg, L. W. 1990. Inhibition of cancer by minor nutrient constituents in the diet. Proc Nutri Soc (Jul) 49(2):173-83.

2. "Since then, two *phytochemicals* (substances found in plants)..."
Michnovicz, J. J., and H. L. Bradlow. 1991. Altered estrogen metabolism and excretion in humans following consumption of indole-3 carbinol, Nutr Cancer 16(1):59-66.
Stroh, M. 1992. Inside Broccoli: A Weapon Against Cancer. Sci News 141:183.

Garlic
Page 6

1. "Garlic has been used as a folk remedy throughout the world..."
Raj, K. P., and R. M. Parmar. 1977. Garlic—condiment and medicine, Ind Drugs 15:205-10.

Page 7

2. "In modern times, animal and laboratory experiments have shown..."
Pizzorno, J., and M. Murray. 1986. *A Textbook of Natural Medicine.* Seattle: Bastyr University Publications.

3. "These compounds may also be effective at fighting bacterial infection..."
Pizzorno, J., and M. Murray. 1986. *A Textbook Of Natural Medicine.* Seattle: Bastyr University Publications.

4. "The National Cancer Institute, the United States Department of..."
Weisberger, A. S., and J. Pensky. 1958. Tumor inhibition by a sulfhydryl-blocking agent related to an active principle of garlic (*Allium sativum*), Cancer Research, 18:1301-08.

Lau, B. H., T. Yamaski, D. S. Gridley. 1991. Garlic compounds modulate macrophage and T-lymphocyte functions. Mol Biother (Jun) 3(2):103-07.

5. "The white blood cells of people who eat garlic..."
Quillin, P. 1994 *Beating Cancer with Nutrition.* Tulsa, Okla.: Nutrition Times Press, Inc.

Carotenoid-rich Foods
Page 8
1. "Carotenoids contain *antioxidants* that may stimulate the immune system..."
Burton, G. W., and K. U. Ingold. 1984. Beta-carotene: an unusual type of antioxidant. Science 11 (May) 224(4649):569-73.

2. "Many studies have reported a relationship between low risk for cancer and..."
American Institute for Cancer Research Information Series, revised Nov. 1991. *The Cancer Process.*

3. "Additionally, beta-carotene is transformed into retinoic acid..."
Harvard Health Letter, April 1995.

Yogurt
Page 9
1. "Some animal and laboratory studies have shown that yogurt..."
Shahani, K. M., et al. 1977. Natural antibiotic activity of *Lactobacillus acidophilus* and *bulgaricus.* Cult Dairy Prod J, 12:8-11.

Gilbert, J. P., et al. 1983. Viricidal Effects of *Lactobacillus* and yeast fermentation. Appl Env Microbiol 46(2):452-58.

2. "Lactobacillus, one of the active cultures found in yogurt..."
Quillin, P. 1994. *Beating Cancer with Nutrition.* Tulsa, Okla.: Nutrition Times Press, Inc.

Conge, G. A., et al. 1980. Comparative effects of a diet enriched in live or heated yogurt on the immune system of the mouse. Reprod Nutr Dev 20(4A):929-38.

3. "The National Cancer Institute has determined that some malignant tumors..."
Balch, P. A., and J. F. Balch. 1992. *Prescriptions for Cooking and Dietary Wellness.* Greenfield, Wis.: P. A. P. Publ. Inc.

van't Veer, P., et al. 1989. Consumption of fermented milk products and breast cancer: a case-control study in the Netherlands. Cancer Res (Jul 15) 49(14):4020-23.

4. "Yogurt also provides important nutrients such as vitamins B6, B12, niacin..."
Pizzorno J., and M. Murray. 1993. *A Textbook of Natural Medicine.* Seattle: Bastyr University Publications.

Beans
Page 10
1. "Most importantly for cancer survivors, beans contain several compounds..."
Kennedy, A. R. 1995. The evidence for soybean products as cancer preventive agents. J Nutr (Mar) 125 suppl:733s-73s.

2. "*Isoflavones* block the entry of estrogen into cells, which may reduce..." Kennedy, A. R. 1995. The evidence for soybean products as cancer preventive agents. J Nutr (Mar) 125 suppl:733s-73s.

Page 11
3. "*Phytosterols* slow the reproduction of cells in the large intestine..."
Janezic, A. A., and A. V. Rao. 1992. Dose-dependent effects of dietary phytosterol on epithelial cell proliferation of the murine colon. Food Chem Toxicol (Jul) 30:7.

4. "*Saponins* are thought to interfere with

the process by which DNA..."
Nutrition Action Healthletter, April 1994.

Soybeans
Page 11
1. "Some scientists believe that differences in soy consumption explain..."
Cassidy, A., S. Bingham, K. D. Setchell. 1994. Biological effects of a diet of soy protein rich in isoflavones on the menstrual cycle of premenopausal women. Am J Clin Nutr (Sept) 60(3):333-40.

Page 12
2. "Because tumors need a great deal of blood to survive..."
Fotsis, T., et al. 1993. Genistein, a dietary derived inhibitor of in vitro angiogenesis. Proc Natl Acad Sci USA 1 (Apr) 90(7):2690-94.

4. "Soybeans also contain protease inhibitors, which some studies show..."
Messina, M. and S. Barnes. 1991. The role of soy products in reducing risk of cancer. J Natl Cancer Inst 17 (Apr) 83(8):541-46.

5. "And finally, *isoflavins*—which are prominent in soybeans..."
Wei, H., et al. 1993. Inhibition of tumor promoter-induced hydrogen peroxide formation in vitro and in vivo by genistein. Nutr Cancer 20(1):1-12.

Citrus Fruit
Page 13
1. "Cells in the immune system, including T cells..."
Baso, T. K. 1983. The significance of ascorbic acid, thiamin, and retinol in cancer. Int J Vit Nutr Res (suppl) 24:105-17.
Hanck, A. 1983. Vitamin C and cancer. Int J Vit Nutr Res (suppl) 24:87-104.

2. "Flavonoids may also hamper the ability of hormones to bind to cells..."
Harvard Health Letter, April 1995.

3. "Studies conducted both in laboratories and with human stbjects..."
National Research Council. 1982. *Diet, Nutrition, and Cancer.* Washington, D.C.: National Academy Press.

4. "Vitamin C is also essential for healthy gums, teeth, bones..."
Simone, C.B. 1992. *Cancer and Nutrition.* Garden City, New York: Avery Publishing Group, Inc.

5. "*Limonene* is a phytochemical found in citrus fruits that accelerates..."
Gould, M. N., et al. 1994. Limonene chemoprevention of mammary carcinoma induction following direct in situ transfer of v-Ha-ras. Cancer Res (Jul 1) 54(13):3540-43.

6. "*Terpenes* are believed to increase those enzymes known to break down..."
Simone, C. B. 1992. *Cancer and Nutrition.* Garden City, New York: Avery Publishing Group, Inc.

Fiber-Rich Foods
Page 14
1. "Studies in 1960 of the Bantu tribe of rural South Africa..."
Simone, C.B. 1992. *Cancer and Nutrition.* Garden City, New York: Avery Publishing Group, Inc.

2. "Fiber acts to speed the passage of food through the gastrointestinal..."
Burkitt, D. P. 1978. Colonic-rectal cancer: fiber and other dietary factors. Am J Clin Nutr 31 (Oct) Suppl: S56-S64.

3. "One study found that women who had two or fewer bowel movements..."
Howe, G. R., et al. 1990. Dietary factors and risk of breast cancer: combined analysis of 12 case-controlled studies. J Natl Cancer Inst 4 (Apr) 82(7):561-69.

4. "A Dutch study, which evaluated women on the basis of grain intake..."
van't Veer, P., et al. 1990. Dietary fiber, beta-carotene, and breast cancer: results from a case control study, Int J Cancer 45:825-28.

Page 15
5. "It has been shown that fiber may have a cancer-preventing effect on..."
van't Veer, P., et al. 1990. Dietary fiber, beta-carotene, and breast cancer: results from a case control study, Int J Cancer 45:825-28.

Howe, G. R., et al. 1990. Dietary factors and risk of breast cancer. J Natl Cancer Inst 4 (Apr) 82(7):561-69.

Fish
Page 15
1. "*Omega-3 fatty acids* found in some fish seem to play a significant role..."
Hamilton, E. N., E. N. Whitney, F. S. Sizer. 1991. *Nutrition Concepts and Controversies,* 5th Ed. Saint Paul, Minn. West Publ. Co.

Page 16
2. "Numerous studies have shown that omega-3 fatty acids may also reduce..."
Simone, C. B. 1992. *Cancer and Nutrition.* Garden City, New York: Avery Publishing Group, Inc.

3. "It has been shown that fish oil may interfere with the production..."
Austin, S., and C. Hitchcock, *Breast Cancer: What You Should Know (But May Not Be Told) About Prevention, Diagnosis, and Treatment.* Rocklin, Calif.: Prima Publishing Co.

4. "Breast cancer patients often produce too much PGE2, which hinders..."
Baxevanis, C. N., et al. 1993. Elevated prostaglandin E2 production by monocytes is responsible for the depressed level of natural killer and lymphokine-activated killer cell function in patients with breast cancer. Cancer 15 (Jul) 72(2): 491-501.

Mushrooms
Page 17
1. "There is evidence that shiitake, maitake and reishi..."
Chihara, G., et al. 1987. Antitumor metas-tasis—inhibitory activities of *lentinan* as an immunomodulator: an overview. Cancer Dect Prev Suppl 1:423-43.

2. "Some researchers believe polysaccharides may activate *macrophages*..."
Wang, H. X., et al. 1995. Immunomodulatory and antitumor activi-ties of a polysaccharide-peptide complex from a mycelial culture of *Tricholoma sp.,* a local edible mushroom. Life Sci 9 (Jun) 57(3):269-81.

3. "One study of maitake mushrooms showed..."
Quillin, P. 1994. *Beating Cancer with Nutrition.* Tulsa, Okla.: Nutrition Times Press, Inc.

4. "The shiitake contains *lentinan,* an antivi-ral substance..."
Baxevanis, C. N., et al. 1993. Elevated prostaglandin E2 production by monocytes is responsible for the depressed levels of nat-ural killer and lymphokine-activated killer cell function in patients with breast cancer. Cancer 15 (Jul) 72(2):491-501.

NUTRIENTS THAT PROMOTE GOOD HEALTH
Fat—A Littler Goeas a long Way
Page 25
1. "Cancers of the breast, prostate, and colon, as well as obesity..."
Balch, P. A., and J. F. Balch. 1992. *Prescription for Cooking and Dietary Wellness.* Greenfield, Wis.: P. A. P. Publ. Inc.

2. "A widely publicized 1992 study reported that there is no link..."
American Institute for Cancer Research Newsletter, Summer 1993. Issue 40.

3. "While excess fat doesn't cause cancers, it may promote..."
Hamilton, E. N., E. N. Whitney, F. S. Sizer. 1991. *Nutrition Concepts and Controversies,* 5th Ed. Saint Paul, Minn.: West Publ. Co.

Page 26
4. "Finally, it has been shown that a low-fat diet may enhance..."
American Institute for Cancer Research Newsletter, Summer 1994.

5. "In both animals and humans, a low-fat diet seems to improve cell..."
Quillin, P. 1994. *Beating Cancer with Nutrition.* Tulsa, Okla.: Nutrition Times Press, Inc.

Vitamins—Necessary for Life and Growth
Page 28
1. "Nobel Prize–winning scientist Linus Pauling found that vitamin C..."
Balch, P. A., and J. F. Balch. 1992. *Prescription for Cooking and Dietary Wellness.* Greenfield, Wis.: P. A. P. Publ. Inc.

Page 29
2. "Fruit and vegetable intake, and most notably vitamin C intake..."
Howe, G. R., et al. Dietary factors and risk of breast cancer: combined analysis of 12 case-controlled studies. J Nat Cancer Inst 4 (Apr) 82(7):561-69.

3. "It is believed that good nutrition decreases recovery time..."
Hamilton, E. N., E. N. Whitney, F. S. Sizer. 1991. *Nutrition Concepts and Controversies,* 5th Ed. Saint Paul, Minn.: West Publ. Co.
Page 30

4. "Calcium may have some preventive value related to colon cancer..."
Harvard Health Letter, April 1995.

5. "Malignancies may be more common in people who have reduced..."
Rosenfeld, I. 1995. *Doctor, What Should I Eat?* New York: Random House, Inc.

6. "Selenium seems to promote antioxidant activities..."
Barnard, N. D. 1990. *The Power of Your Plate.* Summertown, Tenn.: Book Publishing Co.

INDEX

Super Foods.

P. 5

18 (honorable mentions)

Water

P. 19

Protein

P. 20-22, 23, 24

Carbohydrates

P. 24

Fat

P.

Vitamins

P.

Minerals

P.